The
Autistic
Mom

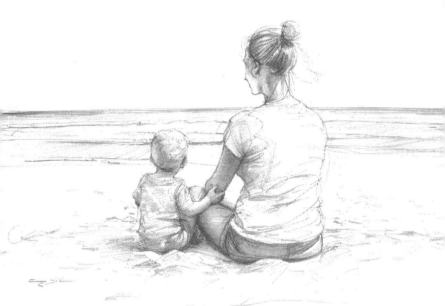

J. Whalley

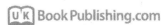 Book Publishing.com

Editing, design, typesetting and publishing by UK Book Publishing

www.ukbookpublishing.com

ISBN: 978-1-916572-95-9

The
Autistic
Mom

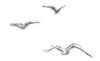

NOTES FROM THE AUTHOR

Throughout this book I will often refer to myself, and other people with **Autism Spectrum Condition (ASC)** and/or **Attention Deficit Hyperactivity Disorder (ADHD)**, as 'we' or 'us'. However, I do not wish to generalise anyone with these conditions.

The topic of this book is endless, and I could discuss it forever, so I have had to choose to write about what is most important to me, my experiences, my opinions and what I have gauged – via my peers and through research – is most important to other autistic people and those with ADHD, and their families. I am aware that as, just like EVERY human being, ALL autistic people and/or people with ADHD are different to the next and we all experience life differently and identify differently. Some may not agree with what I have written or would have liked other issues highlighted. I do not mean to cause any offence, and welcome, and would genuinely appreciate, any feedback on this via the contact details provided at the end of the book.

Abbreviations used throughout this book:

ASC   Autism Spectrum Condition

ADHD   Attention Deficit Hyperactivity Disorder

NT   Neurotypical: people living with a brain that functions in a similar way to most other people

ND   Neurodivergent: people living with a brain that processes, learns and/or behaves differently to what is considered typical

SEN   Special Education Needs

SLT   Speech and Language Therapist

OT   Occupational Therapist

I am different but not less.

Dr. Temple Grandin

*Inspirational Author and
Autism Advocate*

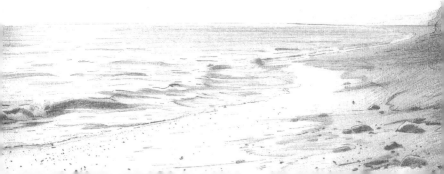

CONTENTS

Jude

You're my magic.
Always be yourself.
Always be happy.
Mummy loves you the most in the whole world.

Shaun

I did it! I know you've not always understood
why I had to do this but thanks for giving
me the space to do so. I love you.

Dr Ryan – thank you for always calling when
you said you would and for doing your best
to guide me over the last 4 years!

Nurse Stephen Burrows – thank you for 'getting
it' and listening to me ramble on in every
review, you're amazing at your job and much
appreciated. Alongside your colleague Dr Johnson
and all he has done for people with ADHD.

Lastly, to all the parents/carers of neurodivergent children, to all the people who work to really support these children, and to all those who struggle with ASC/ADHD or mental health issues – PLEASE KEEP MOVING FORWARD, PLEASE KEEP BEING STRONG. YOU ARE NOT ALONE.

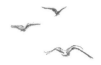

A FEW WORDS FOR THE 'DOUBTERS'

In general, I hope this is a positive read, I'm a big believer in positive thinking and distancing myself from negativity. However, it is a fact that as ASC and in particular ADHD, gain more public awareness, there is a part of society that just don't 'get it'. They just think it's a new trend, a bandwagon that people are jumping on, or they don't believe in the conditions being real at all. Some think it's just another word for 'naughty' kids, spoilt adults or people looking for excuses.

Public comment from charity
ADHD UK October 2023:

ADHD is not fashionable and trivialising it as such is an outrageous smear on the adults and children with a diagnosis. ADHD was only recognised in this country

in the year 2000 for children and in the year 2008 for adults. So, of course, there is a substantial overhang of undiagnosed people coming forward. The increase in talking about ADHD and diagnosis is not fashion. It is not social contagion. It is a result of a failure of diagnosis and care over decades.

Some older generations (and some just plain ignorant people) do not understand the developments of ASC and ADHD. I have often heard the likes of "we didn't have these labels in my day, and we've done ok".

To this I simply say that not having these labels didn't work either because our country is in a mental health epidemic that grows each year, all our prisons are over capacity and alcohol and drug addiction levels are at an all-time high. Past generations had insane asylums and inhumane treatments which didn't work out too great either!

There have been many, many issues throughout history that people didn't understand at the time that are now cemented within our society. There have also been many new conditions and diseases discovered over time and so much progress made within the medical world so it's helpful to keep an open mind. For example, Postpartum Depression (also known as Postnatal Depression) wasn't officially recognised until 1994 when thousands of women have suffered with this for centuries. Some can struggle with this more severely than others and there is no explanation.

I think we can all agree that we live in a VERY different world now to the one in which older generations did – one in which it isn't easy for NT people to cope with the increasing pressures of modern life, so for ND people it's much, much harder because to put pressure on to an already overwhelmed mind becomes unbearable with time. We are ALL completely overloaded with information from social media, the press and television today, and fed the narrative that we should be able to do it all and do it perfectly, as well as having to cope with the continuous negative world developments of our time. If you can live happily without struggles, you're one of the lucky few; for many it's impossible. The communities we live in are also drastically different to what they once were.

Unless you know someone with ASC and/or ADHD you most likely know little about the conditions. Admittedly (and ashamedly but I'm just being brutally honest) I, before having my son, had no clue about either and naively believed that an autistic child was probably just 'naughty' and a child with ADHD was mostly an excuse for poor discipline. I also thought that any parent I had seen publicly bringing focus to the fact their child had either condition was looking for sympathy and attention. Genuinely, I'm embarrassed that my past self was so ignorant; however, this does reflect a part of society which I hope to help educate.

The ONLY way our world will get better is if we educate ourselves and teach our children better. You may not think that you need to be educated or want to be, but there is no doubt that you will have opinions, even unconsciously, because of your upbringing or the world we live in, that are helpful to nobody and only feed into negativity, of which nothing good results.

Just because
you're taught that
something's right
and everyone
believes it's right,
doesn't make it right.

Mark Twain

Historical Writer and Lecturer

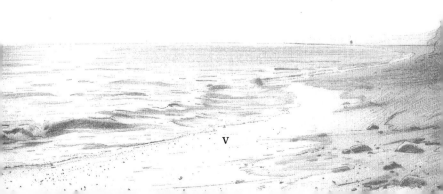

INTRODUCTION

To any NT readers – please keep in mind that I have created this book using my ND mind and this may be noticeable to you in the way it is written. There have been times, during working on this, that I have been struggling with my mental health or going through difficulties which again may affect the way in which I have written; however, I felt it important to be as transparent and honest as possible during these times in the hope that this will help others in similar situations.

This book has taken three years to complete – it was never an option to give up as I felt strongly that I had to write this as it contains all of the information that would have been helpful when I was thrust onto this rollercoaster. There is A LOT of information included and I have tried my best to keep it as easy to read and follow as possible. Also given my nature and strong sense of injustice, there are MANY current social issues that are very important to me, such as education, poverty, healthcare, and homelessness; however, this isn't the topic of my book, so I apologise if I veer off topic at points – I have tried not to.

A lot of the information regarding research/statistics/ policies etc. is taken from the UK, but I believe the essence of the book can be understood and relatable wherever you live in the world.

At the age of 38 I was officially diagnosed with both **Autistic Spectrum Condition** and **Attention Deficit Hyperactivity Disorder** which had been overlooked my entire life. On the outside I'm a 'normal' person, I don't 'look' any different to anyone else, but I have ALWAYS 'felt' different, and I now KNOW that is because my brain works differently to most other people's. Thankfully, I have found a way to care for myself and be positive, and I want to help others in similar circumstances do the same. I am also an 'Autistic Mom', meaning that I am a mother who is autistic AND I have a child who is autistic. I have experienced a wide scale of these conditions from both sides, and I want to help others using what I have learned.

Most readers don't know me, and this book isn't just for people to read about me alone. The personal information I have shared has been done so to help others, particularly other females (the reason for which I will explain), who feel or have felt, the same as I have/do and who have experienced similar things. I also hope to help anyone I can to understand the reality of living with ASC and ADHD. Whilst I'm very aware that there has recently been an 'overload' of information in the media/on social media with regards to ADHD, this journey of mine has been ongoing for almost six years so it is important to me that people understand this isn't about me jumping on any bandwagon.

There are VASTLY different levels (for want of a better word) of ASC and ADHD – the term 'spectrum' is used for this reason. Also, these two conditions can often coincide with other diagnoses and/or disabilities which differ greatly to those I or my son have or do experience. However, I am certain that at least some of the information in this book will be relatable and helpful to all people who read it, especially those within our ND communities, in whatever context.

I would like to make it clear that in my opinion being autistic and/or having ADHD is not an excuse for 'naughty' behaviour (I believe no child is just 'naughty', ALL behaviour is some form of communication from a child); however, allowances do need to be made at times for those who live with these conditions (both adults and children). Believe me when I say we do try, from childhood, to understand and communicate like people want us to, but sometimes it's just physically impossible.

Hopefully as I explain further, more people will be able to understand just how debilitating it can sometimes be to live within a society that is not made for us and does not understand us, and we often don't understand ourselves. These conditions are very difficult at times and our behaviour or communication may sometimes reflect this struggle.

ASC and ADHD are lifelong neurological conditions which must be accepted much like other medical conditions. People with ASC and/or ADHD are born as they are, there is no other way to explain that – it is not a choice, and it is not something we learn. However, this does not HAVE to limit or stigmatise those of us with these conditions. With the right information, support, treatments, mindset, and environments we CAN, and many do, live fulfilling, happy lives. Those of us with ASC and/or ADHD do have to learn to live alongside NT people; HOWEVER, NT people (and the NT world) also must learn to live alongside us as we are – ND. We are both needed, and we are both here and that isn't going to change, and neither should it.

There are many, many people who have lived, or still live, undiagnosed like I did, and many who have had much harder experiences than I have. I'm not a victim, life isn't always easy, more difficult for some than others, and I've learned we must help ourselves. Nothing and nobody will knock on your door and make you happy or help you figure things out. Nobody knows you better than yourself. If you stay strong and learn to understand yourself and love yourself, you CAN help yourself live your happiest life.

> "The most important relationship in your life is the one you have with yourself. Because no matter what happens, you will always be with yourself."
>
> DIANE VON FURSTENBURG – Fashion House Icon

To the parents/carers of children with ASC and/or ADHD reading who feel alone and I know at the beginning of their journey are completely overwhelmed, and have no idea how to best support their child or what this means for them, their families, and the rest of their lives – I hope this book gives you some positive perspective and advice that you can use in your daily lives. Being autistic and/or having ADHD does not have to be a negative **disability** but can always be a **different ability**. If there is support in place then, like physically disabled people who often have accessibility needs to be able to do certain things, we can be the much-needed members of society that we are. Remember we're ALL different whether we're ND or not, and we all have difficulties of some kind, there is no 'perfect' human being.

The more awareness raised, and knowledge learned will only help the diagnosed and undiagnosed children and adults living around us to be accepted and understood for who they are and for what they can achieve; I want to be a part of this growing conversation and an advocate for the ASC and ADHD communities. With regards to ASC alone, it is estimated that there are 700,000 people in the UK with the condition – this cannot be ignored.

Lastly, I truly hope that this book will help anyone who feels alone, feels different, feels lost and/or suspects that they, or someone they know, has ASC and/or ADHD, to navigate their way through their difficulties to live positively and that it helps EVERYONE understand us better.

What's dangerous is not to evolve

Jeff Bezos

Founder and CEO of Amazon

AUTISM SPECTRUM CONDITION AND ATTENTION DEFICIT HYPERACTIVITY DISORDER

ASC and ADHD are neurological conditions which are, thankfully, slowly but surely being brought to attention as more knowledge is discovered and awareness is being raised.

ASC is a lifelong condition that affects how a person makes sense of the world, processes information and relates to other people.

ADHD is a lifelong condition that can affect a person's attention, concentration, hyperactivity, and impulsivity that interferes with their functioning.

Both conditions affect people in different ways and in varying degrees.

Research shows that autistic brains have reduced connectivity between different areas within the brain and that ADHD brains do not produce enough, or process, the natural chemical dopamine which affects the way several areas of the brain work. Over time we will continue to learn more as the conditions continue to be studied and treated.

As more is learned of these conditions, many children and adults are being diagnosed. Historically females have been overlooked as generally more males than females are diagnosed. With regards to ASC, just 30 years ago the rates were thought to be 10:1 but now we know it is more like 2:1. We also now know that females are actually just better at 'masking' their ND traits and copying others to 'fit in' (I learned from a young age how I was 'supposed' to be and did that rather than being myself). Females are naturally more socially motivated so from childhood autistic girls tend to copy those around us and in turn we don't show our true selves; females also tend to be less hyperactive and internalise their symptoms, all of which means our symptoms go unnoticed, by professionals and even parents (particularly for those from older generations who grew up when less was known about these conditions).

In general, male and female brains are different, for example men often have higher levels of the natural chemical serotonin which explains why they don't struggle as much with getting stuck in negative thought cycles or obsessive-compulsive behaviours as women do. Research has shown that the blood flow to the prefrontal cortex of the brain is higher in females than in males which helps them have more self-control. So, whilst females can 'mask' their symptoms better than males, we are usually struggling a lot more on the inside. The problem with this is that as we get older the energy and effort it takes to do this takes a huge toll on us both physically and mentally and it's practically impossible to sustain without causing real problems. It is estimated that one in four women with undiagnosed ADHD attempt to take their own lives and that there are currently, at the very least, 35,000 undiagnosed females in the UK who are autistic and unaware, struggling through life every single day most likely thinking they're losing their minds – they're not – and I hope I can help some to understand this. They will often suffer with worsening mental and physical health, addiction, poor relationships, problems with their career, debt, vulnerability, and low self-esteem to name a few common issues.

Of course, as we all get older our stresses, responsibilities and the demands of life get harder, and for women our hormones fluctuate; this pressure can lead to our symptoms becoming more overwhelming and harder to control as we struggle to continue to 'cope' with them. It's normally at this point that mental health issues are diagnosed. If you seek help with being overwhelmed the first thing a doctor will usually say is that you have anxiety/depression. Unless you already have experience or knowledge of ASC and/or ADHD, nobody would think either of these could be the issue. This is the reason most ND women only discover that they have one of these conditions when they have a child who is diagnosed (this was the case for me).

The highest age range for death by suicide in the UK, for both men and women, is between the ages of 45 and 54. The fact that this happens at this point in life is no surprise to me. The pressure of life by this age can often become unbearable, and ND or not some people unfortunately find it just too difficult. This age group also has the highest level of addiction for both drugs and alcohol and at least half of people with addiction issues also have a mental health problem. Whilst men are three times more likely to take their own life, women are more likely to have suicidal thoughts and attempt suicide. The number of women reporting mental health problems has been rising year on year. It is known that a large percentage of ND people turn to substance abuse to 'numb' the overwhelm in their minds because, especially when living undiagnosed, it is an isolating and excruciatingly difficult condition to manage. People in minority groups, such as the LGBTQIA+ community, are more likely to suffer, this is for reasons such as being treated differently because they're not the 'same' as the majority, along with hiding their true selves, which is painful to live with day in day out.

Alongside the fact that it is very common for people with ADHD and/or ASC to suffer with depression and/or anxiety, the conditions often bring physical health issues with them – as yet we don't know why this is. Some examples are: joint problems such as Fibromyalgia (often as a result of being hypermobile), gastrointestinal and digestive issues such as Crohn's Disease, Epilepsy, eating disorders, sleep issues and Tourette's Disorder.

We know, in the UK, that the National Health Service (NHS) is massively overstretched and sadly most GPs are just not trained thoroughly enough with regards to ND (at present) to be able to spot ASC or ADHD as easily as they potentially could, so unless you can afford to see a private specialist/ psychiatrist who specialise in these conditions (which the average person cannot) then you could be stuck in a vicious circle of trying different medications for different mental health issues that ultimately don't help. Again, this was the case for me and like most people I trusted that my GP would have the best resources and that I wouldn't have to turn to researching things myself (luckily, I also had an experienced and proactive NHS therapist who was on the ball).

Receiving a diagnosis, as early as possible, is so crucial to improving the lives of people living with ASC and/or ADHD. I will detail this process from both having a child diagnosed (my son Jude was diagnosed with ASC aged three and ADHD aged eight) and as an adult being diagnosed later in life. Research shows that untreated, misdiagnosed, or undiagnosed ASC and ADHD increases the risk of heart disease, cancer, obesity, diabetes and developmental problems, schizophrenia and suicidal thoughts.

Currently, in the UK, there aren't any different scales on diagnosis – ASC is ASC no matter what level the person is affected, and ADHD is usually ADHD or ADD. However, many of us within the ND community don't agree with this as the needs of one person to the next can differ greatly, which means so can their treatments and support needs. It is believed that there are at least seven different 'types' of ADHD and each type has different medications, supplements and therapy that can help. I have Overfocused ADD for which a mix of stimulant medication and anxiety medication is the most beneficial, BUT it took me several agonising years to discover this – if more effort was focused on support and more training was given to GPs this would not have been the case. Our diagnosis process needs to be more efficient and the knowledge of the scale of differences we have needs to vastly improve so that we can all be treated and helped more individually, efficiently, and beneficially.

In school, children with ASC and/or ADHD need to be provided with, at the very minimum, amendments to their education because they learn differently to their NT peers. A ND child can accomplish a high level of education IF they are given the right tools and support – they won't receive this without a diagnosis. As adults, the sooner we receive a diagnosis, the sooner we can understand ourselves and begin to use treatments, learn to understand ourselves and get support to help us live a happier, healthier life.

In late 2022, there was a debate in parliament in which the UK government was asked to create an emergency fund to deal with the huge waiting lists for ASC and ADHD assessments for both children and adults. They were also asked to review the way in which the NHS manage and record the data from assessments. They were asked for better training for all people involved in working with children, mental health services and local authorities regarding Education Health Care Plans (EHCPs). The inadequate post diagnosis support has also been brought to attention. The current national Autism Strategy says that "we will have made demonstratable progress on reducing diagnosis waiting times and improving diagnosis pathways for children, young people and adults". The fact that this has FINALLY been discussed and taken seriously is positive and I hope a step in the right direction for much needed, overdue change. Thank you to the people who have, and continue, to campaign for this – many who are parents of ND children.

I want to bring a voice to the fact that having ASC and/or ADHD is nothing to be ashamed of. Not many people want a label, or want a label for their child, but getting a diagnosis truly helps you understand yourself. It helps the people around you understand you and gives you access to much needed treatment and support. You can start to LIVE your life and have a more positive future. Being autistic and/or having ADHD does not have to hold you or your child back.

As previously mentioned, there is definite progress with regards to awareness of ASC and ADHD, there are also positive changes as the world naturally evolves. Here is a quick example that was a very common occurrence in past years; I recently met a lady who was in her late seventies who was telling me that sadly her son had passed away recently in his fifties. Her son had lived in supported housing as he was autistic and had some other difficulties, such as he was profoundly deaf, but he wanted to live, like most adults do, independently from his parents. We then got to discussing ASC and she told me that when her son was born in the seventies, the hospital had told her and her husband that they would be best to leave their child with them as he would be "too hard to look after" and that they should "go and enjoy their lives". This was only 50 years ago – essentially not that long ago and that would never even be thought of now let alone said. Just imagine what will change for the better in the next 10, 20, 30 plus years...try to remember this if you ever feel hopeless or worry about the future for your child.

Side note – this family did indeed look after their son well, although difficult at times due to their generation and lack of knowledge and support, and their son lived HIS life happily.

Being born ND is the luck of the draw, to put it bluntly it is what it is, and it cannot be prevented. As these are not visible conditions, they are not given the same care and compassion as a physical disability. They may be seen as a poor excuse or a weakness. This is, at best, ignorant. Please KNOW that if someone has a diagnosis (or are on the pathway towards one or really need to be) they should be supported accordingly, they have a genuine neurological condition, it is not something that can be faked, and it is certainly not easy to get a diagnosis in any respect, so if someone has one it's because it is necessary.

Humanity
evolves thanks to
people who think
differently and
discover new ways
hidden from the
majority.

L. William Ross

Author and ADHD Expert

Part One

My Story

MY MILENNIAL CHILDHOOD

Every generation learns from the last and hopefully does better. The way of the world and how we are brought up is not our choice, but it does affect the rest of our lives and we can choose better as we grow up and for our own children. My generation was for the most part raised by younger parents, parents who put emphasis on marriage even when they were not happy marriages, and parents who believed that children should be seen and not heard.

I didn't have the happiest childhood, I always knew I was different somehow and I always felt lonely, I didn't come from a close-knit loving family, and I didn't have great support, my family is very small, there wasn't a lot of close aunties, uncles, and cousins around. My earliest memory is of domestic violence against my mum, when I was four years old. However, during my younger years I somehow always knew there was more out there for me.

I've always been self-aware, independent and strong, and this has helped me throughout my life. The strongest people you meet will always have a story; they are who they are because of their experiences. If you've had a difficult childhood, been around domestic abuse or just never felt loved, do not think that you must continue the same pattern. You can move on, there is always a way to undo the behaviour you have been privy to, and your past does not have to be your future.

Like many children from my generation, I come from a 'broken home'. When I was five years old my mum married a man, who even at such a young age I instinctively disliked. My experience with him has meant that I have never been able to stand any kind of controlling man (which was reinforced following my first relationship as I detail in Relationships Section One), and I have never relied on a man – or anyone else in fact. Over the years I was often told how I should be grateful to him for "putting a roof over my head" when I wasn't his child and how I was "loved but not liked" – difficult for a child who always felt on the outside anyway. Eventually at age 18 I finally got my own home and never looked back.

My mum and I have never had a 'typical' mother/daughter relationship. My mum is the only person who has known me my whole life and has always been in my life, but we just don't have a close bond. Everyone is different, it is what it is, it can often be a difficult relationship, that of a mother and daughter; I'm sure there are many psychological reasons behind this, most girls/women I know have experienced this and still do, but all we can do is accept people for who they are and try and do better for our own relationships with our children – especially given all the knowledge now available to us that our parents didn't have. I had a very close bond with my nanna (my mum's mum) but sadly she died when I was just nine years old. Like a lot of children from single parent families (which I was for the first five years of my life) I spent a lot of time with my grandparents, and I adored my nanna. She showered me with the praise and affection that I craved (something all children need and deserve). To this day she is the only person I have ever been shown unconditional maternal love by.

I have two siblings (one sister, one brother) who are seven and nine years younger than me respectively. They both had, and still do have, quite a different relationship with our mum, and I've genuinely never envied this, I've always wanted the best for them; I was a very parental part of their childhood as I was the oldest and spent a lot of time 'babysitting' them. I adored my younger siblings, and they were the only source of happiness for me at home – even now my sister is the closest person to me except my husband and son.

Looking back on my childhood is just unhappy, I was sad and lonely. Any chance I got I would be in my bedroom alone reading, writing, or sleeping. I LOVED to read, books were my escape to other places, families, friends, and experiences. I never sat with my parents to watch TV or to just be together as a family and I was never asked. I ate meals with them, but I soon learned to look after myself and just avoided being around them as much as possible – if they were home, I was in my bedroom or out. If I had the chance I always liked to sleep out, other homes were just so much more relaxed and I didn't have the responsibilities I did at my own.

The only good childhood memories I have are from our family holidays and still now I LOVE a holiday more than the average person – although it does take a huge amount of planning and preparation for myself and my son, but it's worth it. On holiday everyone is generally more relaxed, laid back; you often go out for meals (I'm a big foodie) and the sun is always shining, which I love. As a child on holiday, however, I did notice, because of being around so many other families, that my family was often different. My parents weren't loving in the ways that other parents were, I wasn't being wrapped up in a towel and cuddled after a day at the pool, but this is something that I just accepted and have made peace with over the years and it's the total opposite of the parent I am to my son.

Once I moved out of the family home, for years I rarely had contact with my mum other than about my siblings or if I desperately needed help as she was the only person I had to ask, and I never spoke to my stepdad again. They divorced when I was 21. I would love to be able to speak to my younger self to tell her to keep going, that it won't always be this way, to stay strong and to be positive. To really think about the life you want, and achieve it and that you will be loved for who you are. You will be happy. You are not less than ANYONE. Just be yourself.

I had a sporadic relationship with my biological dad throughout my childhood. He had a history of violence against women and has his own issues; by his own admittance he cannot commit to a stable relationship with me (or my son), so I no longer have any contact with him and haven't seen him properly for over 20 years. It genuinely doesn't bother me at all that I've never had a positive father figure in my life and I don't miss what I've never had. Surprisingly, I don't feel like I have any 'daddy issues' that have affected my relationships other than the fact that I won't stand being controlled in any way and that I'm not someone who NEEDS a man in their life – but I don't think these are bad 'issues' to have.

Looking over my background, alone and in therapy, it's been good for me to think about how I have grown up to be as trusting and self-assured as I have. The whole 'nature vs nurture' topic is something that has always been very interesting to me. How some people's childhoods, and how they are raised or what they have experienced, can really impact their adult lives in a negative way and others move forward and almost use it to their advantage. You often get siblings who are brought up in exactly the same home, with exactly the same parents, grow up to be entirely different.

To all parents – remember children aren't children for long and what you put in you get out even when they grow up, they will remember things you don't, and this plays a huge part in the rest of their lives. You can't put in little effort in the younger years and expect a great relationship or love and support as you get older.

The true character of a society is revealed in how it treats its children

Nelson Mandela

Renowned Activist and Politician

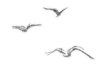

MY SCHOOL
EXPERIENCE

M y school days don't hold many good memories either; everyone says, "you'll miss it when you leave" and "they're the best days of your life" – this is not true for me and never was. Right from the start it just wasn't easy for me and from the day I started secondary school in 1995 I wanted it to be the day I left. Knowing now that I am autistic and have ADHD that makes a lot of sense, but back then my conditions were never picked up on – ADHD was only officially recognised in the year 2000. When I had my ASC assessment in 2022, I was told that ASC was known of in the nineties but only in those visibly, severely affected by the condition so because I hit all my milestones, could walk, and talk etc like my peers and was intelligent, I just didn't stand out. However, these days every nursery and school setting have a checklist for each child and if there are certain issues or areas of concern they are flagged up for further assessment. This alone shows how far we have come in the last 20 plus years, but there is still a long way to go including the fact that many children (especially girls) with ASC and/or ADHD still go under the radar because they may not present with 'typical symptoms', and education staff are not given enough training.

There are so many amazing teachers and school staff who spend their whole careers trying to change the way things are. They advocate for early assessment and intervention because they see first-hand the needs that some children have and what the right support can do. I know most feel like they are 'hitting their heads against a brick wall' trying to get the powers-that-be to listen. Please don't give up – you may not think you're making a difference but as a parent to an autistic child who has attended both mainstream and SEN settings, trust me when I say you do, and our families need you.

When you're in school everything seems so permanent, you don't know what life is like outside of your school years and this can be hard for those who don't fit in to that environment. If you're still in school, please remember this won't always be the case and you will be able to create your own life once you have finished your education – I know it seems endless but just stay strong and do your best.

As I wasn't a happy child, I now know that I didn't come across as particularly nice which probably wasn't much fun to be around (something I didn't realise at the time). A friend I went to school with told me a few years ago that she used to be scared of me and remembers that one day her mum asked her to go to the shop and she saw me outside so turned around and went back home to avoid me. Honestly it blew my mind to learn that this was someone's memory of me, and I was not aware of this at all. I have never been aggressive or violent in my life; however, my mouth has always been smart, and I have always been very defensive. It's no surprise that I never had any 'real' friends – which I'm sure didn't help my school experience. Of course, now knowing what I do I understand that because of ASC I have always found social skills difficult, I also never had the opportunity to learn at home what friendships looked like and how important they are because this was never discussed, and my parents rarely socialised with us. I simply didn't (and to be honest still don't) naturally understand social relationships and all the unwritten rules like most NT people do.

I've read many autistic people say that they feel like everyone else except them were given the handbook on how to behave or how to socialise, and it is exactly like that for me. In school ALL the other girls seemed to just know what to say to each other and how to make friends, whereas

I had to try and learn from watching them, always trying to catch up, and it always felt so awkward. Although I've learned more with time and am used to it, it still does. I was friendly with a couple of girls who lived close by and they're still in my small group of friends now, but mostly the girls I did "hang around" with in secondary school always seemed to be the same kind, not quite bullies – I have always hated any kind of bullying – but the kids who were not the nicest and usually up to no good. The kids who smoked, didn't pay attention in lessons, and answered back to teachers etc. I was drawn to these personalities as a child and I'm still not sure why because I was never a 'naughty' kid. Thankfully, I have, however, always had my own mind and would never have been pushed in to doing something I really didn't want to do. I have also always had my own way, done my own thing, I was never concerned with looking like everyone else like most of the girls were, a quality I still have now.

I also always felt more comfortable in the company of boys; even now I think there is less pressure and what you see is what you get in male friendships. However, I was not interested in the boys at school in any other way than friendship whatsoever, which again was different to most other girls my age. While they were boy mad and some even having sex towards the end of high school, it was the last thing on my mind, and I would not be pressured into it either. I was smitten with the usual teenage idols such as Leonardo DiCaprio and popular boy bands, but real-life boys didn't even hit my radar. I didn't have a proper boyfriend until I was 17. This is an autistic trait I'm glad I have, and my son does too, being strong willed and not following the crowd. I know that some young autistic people, particularly girls, can be led astray quite easily as they try so hard to copy others around them to fit in, which can make them vulnerable and we really need to help children understand that the only way to be truly happy is to be yourself and to be around people with whom they don't have to 'mask' their true selves or be made to do anything they don't want to do.

I would say I mostly just flew under the radar at school. I was always very bright but only interested in learning subjects that I wanted to, such as reading, writing, history, and business studies (which I particularly excelled in). I found it very difficult to concentrate on anything other than my favourite subjects and was easily distracted, I literally couldn't sit still – these I now know are symptoms of ADHD which I'm positive would be picked up on if I was at school now, my school reports literally reel off ADHD traits and were used as part of my ASC and ADHD assessments. Maths I hated and subsequently failed at GCSE; the teacher may as well have been speaking a different language because I couldn't understand a word of what he said. Nowadays, I would most likely have had some extra support with maths for example, and I'm glad that this is commonplace for many children who struggle at school now.

If I could have afforded to, I would have continued with college and university because I really enjoyed learning about the subjects I was interested in (I always wanted to be a journalist), but as I lived alone from a young age, this wasn't possible. If I had had support and guidance, it could have been a different story; however, I genuinely don't wish this to be different because I am more than happy with the life I have now.

I left school in the year 2000 and never really kept in touch with anyone at all, except the girls I already knew. I never particularly 'fell out' with anyone, it was just once school was taken out of the equation there was no desire to keep in touch. Twelve years of being around the same people and I had made no real attachments at all.

Don't confuse a season
for a lifetime.

Even your trials have
an expiration date.

You will grow, life
will change, things
will work out.

Brittney Moses

Author and Mental Health Advocate

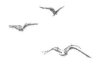

WORK AND NEURODIVERGENCE

For me, employment has been a huge rollercoaster, I had 15 jobs over the 14 years, between leaving school and having Jude. This was worked out in my ADHD assessment – I'd never sat and thought about it before, it's just how it was – this was one of the many deciding factors for my diagnosis. Admittedly, I can struggle to take orders from others and as I've mentioned I'm not good with control, especially from people who 90% of the time I think (usually correctly) that I can do a better job than, and I don't take criticism well (common autistic traits). At a young age I mostly worked in customer service roles, as they were the easiest jobs to get, and when you don't naturally have the best social skills this work isn't ideal and was not suitable for me at all, although at the time I didn't know why I struggled. However, once I am engaged, interested, and appreciated, there is nobody who works like me. I always received high praise from my managers/employers but had many issues within my workplaces. For me I found it best to work for myself after having Jude, I know it's impossible for everyone to do that but if you can, I would recommend that to my ND peers – especially if you have a particular interest that you can make into work – you'll then truly enjoy what you do every day and do it better than anyone else.

For several years I worked within social housing which I really did enjoy, and it opened my eyes to many social issues, the impact of which has stayed with me.

People with ADHD, in general, can struggle in the workplace – especially those who are undiagnosed, untreated, and unsupported. Poor timekeeping, inability to focus, hyperactivity, impulsivity, and procrastinating, being just some of the traits we can hold – not exactly the 'ideal' employee. For those (that we know of) with ASC, unemployment rates are almost 80% in the UK – the highest percentage for any disability.

Truly this is such a shame as ND people can offer so much to their employers and colleagues. Accommodations can and should be made for such employees, in the right environment and with understanding employers, we can and do bring a different vision and unique skills that others simply cannot. In fact, there are companies who actively seek to recruit ND staff because of the abilities we can have that are very well suited to specific roles. We have SO much to offer, but many NT workplaces, restrictions, and job interviews, for example, are not the best way to see us shine. If you think about most job vacancy ads, they ask for qualities such as flexibility, teamworking and good communication skills. Of course, for those with ASC these are not skills that we usually possess, through no fault of our own, but that shouldn't mean we can't be employed. Again, widespread awareness, knowledge and further research will improve this.

Recently I was disappointed to listen to a podcast featuring Kim Kardashian (hugely successful entrepreneur and reality star if by any chance you're unaware) whose show I have always been a big fan of, in which she stated that due to her own close family and long-term friendships one of the areas she looks at for potential employees are their relationships. How close they are to their family, how long they have had their friends for etc. From someone who has access to huge resources, seems so open minded and I know does a lot for charitable causes, I was saddened to hear this. But this is an example of the underlying, and unconscious, opinions that people have. If for some reason you're not close to your family that shouldn't go against you, or if you have difficulties in making friends that doesn't mean you won't be an excellent employee.

It is an ongoing part of the UK government's Autism Strategy that employment rates for people with ASC improve in the coming years – after all, there are more autistic adults than autistic children, and all autistic children will grow up to be autistic adults.

Officially for those who cannot work due to these conditions, either short term or long term, there is financial support available; however, they are notoriously difficult for ND people to claim compared to people with physical disabilities. A department of the authority who are supposed to support people in need, have highly insufficient understanding in conditions such as ASC and ADHD and often negatively impact the health conditions of vulnerable people. Again, not good enough from the people who have all the resources possible at the disposal.

Not everything that steps out of line, and thus "abnormal", must necessarily be "inferior".

Dr. Hans Asperger

Historical Autism Pioneer

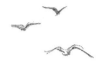

FRIENDSHIPS

One of the hardest things about being autistic is friendships and socialising – one of the known main areas of difficulty in ASC is that of social communication. We usually battle with being consumed in our own worlds but also wanting to have friendships that we see other people have. It is a very lonely place because not many people really know what it's like to be us. We often also have intense interests that most other people don't relate to. However, you do get used to being who you are, and it doesn't mean you can't have friendships and relationships, they're just usually a bit 'different'. The best thing for us to do is to accept that everyone is different and if we're happy in ourselves, remember that we don't have to have a social life like NT people. What makes one person happy doesn't make every other person happy and it doesn't have to. There is no use in comparing ourselves to people who have brains that work completely differently to ours, we would be fighting a losing battle. We don't need to fit in to a mould of something or someone others think we 'should' be, which is very common in people with ASC, and something that took me a long time be comfortable with.

Of course, we can and do have friends and it is important to have connections in your life outside of your family. I also know that it can be much easier for many autistic people to make friends with people online, where there is less pressure or scrutiny, especially in forums with other ND people that you wouldn't have the opportunity to meet in your real life (I list some popular sites that are monitored towards the end of the book, as of course you must be careful within the cyber world especially if you are socially vulnerable).

From a very young age I've chatted to my son about how we're all different and that we should always be nice and kind to others because these are valuable skills to have. I've also always, literally since he was born, set up little playdates for him to allow him to experience being around other children (both ND and NT) having fun so he can understand the positive benefits of socialising. It's proven that having connections with others is good for your mental well-being and overall health. As children get older, they can decide how much and on what terms they want to do this for themselves. Supporting your child to learn these skills and to be a kind and understanding person is a huge part of our job as parents, and I know from my own experience that this will be helpful.

I've always found it difficult to sustain friendships; I rarely 'fall out' with anyone, it's just things naturally grow apart. Another trait I have is that I can be quite black and white;, for example, if someone hurts me or I really don't agree with the way they live their life, I can walk away from the friendship/relationship without a second thought. I am a naturally trusting person but once I lose trust or respect, I am done. This can be a blessing and a curse as can be being brutally honest. I am 100% myself and find it hard to remember that other people aren't as forthright as I am, or that many people are more sensitive or easily offended. More recently as I've found a more positive mindset, I really see when people talk or think negatively, and I just can't be around it.

Given the ADHD part of my personality, I usually get along well with anyone and am not shy, I can hold a conversation with most people in most situations and can often be genuinely interested in them; however, I've never really learned how to move past that point. I know that most people don't understand me, and now having my diagnoses I can see why, because clearly, I have been different my whole life whether I look it or not. I've concluded that it must feel to other people like they can't quite put their finger on what it is that's different about me (even if they're not consciously thinking that) which I guess is understandable. As I previously mentioned, autistic people don't naturally know how to behave in social settings like NT people do. I know that sometimes the way my face sits doesn't fit the situation, and that in some circumstances it feels uncomfortable for me to smile so it's no surprise that I have been told many times over the years that I look unfriendly.

Working and the real world outside of school gave me the chance to meet all different kinds of people and the opportunity for a new kind of social life. As an adult I have always liked 'different' people who dress their own way and have their own opinions; there wasn't much of that in school. In my younger days socialising always involved going to bars/clubs – I have always loved music and dancing. There wasn't any social media then, no camera phones, it wasn't about what you looked like, what you had or where you were from. It makes me sad for young people now that their world revolves around all of that and they're constantly taking pictures and not enjoying the moment, but I understand the world changes. I'm not sure how I would have coped with the pressure they have now, and I have genuinely fun memories of those more carefree times.

When I was 21, I broke up with my boyfriend of three years and lost most of the 'friends' I had because they were all girlfriends of his friends. However, at that age you will always find other young people who want to get out and have a good time and I soon had a circle of people that I would be with all weekend. Some girls, some boys, some I already knew, others new and they were all chilled, down to earth people who just wanted fun, no drama. We didn't talk about anything serious, and I never really saw them outside of going out, so it was easy-going. I always had another side of me that my friends didn't know about and probably didn't care to know about to be honest. I had much more responsibility than them, I bought my own house when I was 21 and most of them still lived with their parents.

During this time, I didn't live a healthy lifestyle at all, I would be out all weekend with barely any sleep, then in the week I would work, go home, eat and sleep and it was like that for three years straight. In the past I have looked back, and thought was I depressed in those days? Because I really didn't have much of a life at all and was always so tired, but I now think that I was just unhealthy and unfulfilled (as I will explain later, I also have two autoimmune diseases which were still undiagnosed at this time as was the fact I had ASC and ADHD). I was at my lowest weight, around seven stone, and really wasn't looking after myself. However, I'm so glad I had that time because I would have hated to be someone who gets older and then thinks they've missed out or that the grass is greener.

Once I was in the social circle I was, I didn't like anyone new getting involved and I now know this is because I am autistic not unfriendly, which as I've mentioned I know some people thought of me. My friend would often say "the more the merrier" and invite someone that I didn't know, and it made me so uncomfortable. They could have been the nicest person in the world, but I just liked what I knew. I also liked going to the same places, I never liked to try anything new. I liked to know the layout, what the music would be like, who the staff were, what the drinks were like and I'm still the same now, it just makes me feel more comfortable. I also don't like to change plans last minute and if someone couldn't make it as planned, I would be really frustrated. When I have spoken with some girls from back then and told them I had been diagnosed, one said "that's why you were always a bit weird" – very unfiltered but I am too, so I like honesty. She told me how I always had "funny little ways"'. It's so strange to hear things like this because I didn't notice any of this at the time, it wasn't until I learned more about ASC and ADHD and looked back that the puzzle started to come together.

As I have explained I didn't have the social skills to build and maintain friendships as a child, so I don't as an adult have the social foundations that many people have from school or college. Although I've always been a positive person and happy within myself, I have never felt like anybody's number one (until my husband and son). I was always on the outside looking in. At home my stepdad always came first, with friends if there were three of us, I was always the odd one out, I was never anyone's first choice or 'best' friend. To this day I wouldn't say I have a 'best' friend. My closest friend lives a five-hour drive away from me so I don't see her often, although we speak regularly; other than that I don't socialise much at all. Writing this book and looking at myself, I've concluded that I've subconsciously chosen not thave many friends because it is easier for me, I don't like to be around people all the time. Also, not many people understand ND people so it's difficult to receive or give what is needed. I know that not many people 'get' me and would say that nobody truly knows ME, even my family who have known me my whole life. This can be hard, but I also enjoy my own company very much and couldn't cope with a hectic social life. Many women also make friends throughout their pregnancies, from antenatal classes or new baby groups etc; however, I lived away from home when I was pregnant, and up until my son was three years old, so all the little groups we were a part of got left behind when we moved back.

Over the years, I've genuinely not understood a lot of friendships I've seen around me, I'm fiercely loyal and it baffles me when I see people talking behind their friends' backs, I just don't get it, this is something else that I'm black and white on – this is something I think that has affected my friendships. I know many people want to be the 'most popular' or have everyone in the world like them, but to me I think if you don't like someone just don't interreact with them or at least don't be fake just so people think you're nice. I also don't understand why there is such fierce competition between other females, I suppose it's always been a part of life, like it's ingrained into girls to hate on their peers instead of supporting and encouraging each other, but it makes no sense. Jealousy is an emotion that helps NOBODY, and we all need to remember (and teach our children, especially girls) that others succeeding doesn't make our chances of succeeding any less, in fact the opposite.

Words by Chimamanda Ngozi Adichie

"We say to girls you can have ambition, but not too much. You should aim to be successful, but not too successful. Otherwise, you will threaten the man.

Because I am female, I am expected to aspire to marriage, I am expected to make my life choices always keeping in mind that marriage is the most important.

Now marriage can be a source of joy, love and mutual support BUT why do we teach girls to aspire to marriage and we don't teach boys the same?

We raise girls to see each other as competitors, not for jobs or for accomplishments (which I think can be a good thing) but for the attention of men.

We teach girls that they cannot be sexual beings in the way that boys are."

Another reason socialising is even more difficult for me now is because I have a child who is autistic; any other autistic parents reading will understand. Raising and supporting an autistic child, especially one who is non-verbal, can be very time consuming. My whole life revolves around my son and that's the way it must be for him to be as happy and settled as he is, and I'm genuinely happiest when I'm with him, I am so grateful to be his mum. Given Jude's needs it's not a case of being able to spontaneously last-minute drop Jude with a family member or friend to play or to stay over. It takes a lot of preparation and planning for everyone involved to make sure Jude's routines are followed and that he is settled in a different environment with someone he is comfortable with. As my son has limited communication/ social skills he doesn't yet have any friends of his own that he has independently chosen so there isn't anywhere he would go for a playdate without me. Also, whoever looks after him needs to be familiar to him and to understand him inside out so they can understand when and what he is communicating.

As an adult I know I have had people try to befriend me, but it gets a bit much for me and I back off, not necessarily because I don't want to be friends with them but because it just doesn't feel natural to me and I don't know how to be in certain situations; it's hard to explain – I know other autistic people will understand this. I also just don't know how people fit in a social life, how does anyone have the energy at the end of the day to go out and socialise?! There have also been people I've met over the years who I would have quite liked to befriend, but I've always been overly aware of other people's thoughts and have never wanted to sound awkward (because that's how I feel) in asking them if they want to meet up, so I just don't, or if one of us does, the busy lives we lead make it hard to schedule and it just gets forgotten about. I do think it gets harder for any woman to make friends as they get older because everyone has their own full lives – careers, children, families, partners etc – and the effort it takes to start and maintain a new friendship usually just isn't possible. It would take someone who really takes the time to get to know me, to really understand me and brings something positive to my life for me to be coaxed out of my bubble.

Now understanding ASC and ADHD, I have done a lot of research to try and understand how social relationships work and to be honest about my diagnoses with the friends/family I have so that people can understand me better. The awareness being raised about ND also helps. One thing about most autistic people is that if you make an effort, and don't let them down, they will be the most loyal, honest and genuine friends you can have. I do know that with the right group there is nothing like being together with other females – only other women understand what it is like to be a woman, to be a mother, a wife, and the many difficulties we face in life – and I do love a girls' night out maybe twice a year which I think is important and I do enjoy, the friends I have understand that I often need to take a timeout alone or do things a certain way.

For a long time, I did struggle with what I thought I 'should' have in the way of friendships as opposed to what I actually wanted. Being diagnosed with and then learning about ASC, I now know that there is nothing 'wrong' with me, I just am who I am and I'm proud of who I am. I give my all to those who are in my life (the only people in my life are those that I have chosen to be) and I am very grateful for what I have. I would also do anything for anyone who needed help. I'm not a jealous person in the slightest and I will trust anyone unless they give me reason not to. All we can do is accept ourselves and remember to always be ourselves because that is the only way to be truly happy. As you get older, I think you naturally accept yourself more and at this point in my life if people don't make an effort with me, I don't give anything either and whoever wants to be in my life will be and those who don't won't. This I am genuinely content with and there are no negative feelings at all. I can sometimes feel that to the people in my life I give more than they do in return, which can be a difficult feeling for me to manage; however, I also am firm in believing that I don't want to stop being who I am because I don't feel I'm getting the same back – I don't give to receive. I don't hold expectations of anyone anymore in that way, something I have got hung up on in the past, and if it really gets to me l now know how to look after myself by taking some time and thinking things through logically.

Each time a woman stands up for herself, without knowing it, possibly without claiming it, she stands up for all women.

Maya Angelou

Author, Poet, Activist

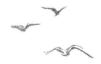

RELATIONSHIPS
– SECTION ONE

From 18 to 21, I had a boyfriend who was a typical 'bad boy'; at a young age many girls are attracted to this kind of person. At first, he was charming as they often are, I think I was probably rebelling a bit seeing him because I had lived in such a strict environment for so long and he was the total opposite of what I was used to. People who know me now would never believe that I put up with what I did from him. I find it can often be the case, people who you think would never stand for such behaviour, surprisingly can do behind closed doors and you would never know.

He soon moved in with me and it was just chaos from the start, constant drama, arguing, jealousy, punching walls and doors, and controlling behaviour. He never actually 'hit' me, but like many people who use domestic violence do, he would push me around, grip me hard or throw things at me. He'd tell me if I left him, he would burn my family's home down when they were asleep, just awful things that I genuinely believed. On one occasion, at his mum's house, there was a pizza delivered and he opened the box and pushed it right in my face, in front of his mum. She was also scared of him so didn't do anything. He was very controlling and so jealous that if another boy even looked in my direction, he would literally start a fight. I absolutely would not condone this kind of behaviour now, living life walking on eggshells is an awful feeling. I can't stand any kind of jealousy or possessiveness or violence. I just won't be around someone who is constantly looking for a fight or an argument, it's no way to live. I genuinely believe that things happen for a reason, and it was a lesson that I'm glad I learned.

I don't know why I got pulled into that situation for so long but, he did have a big close-knit family, so I think being taken in by them initially had something to do with it. Once I was in it, I didn't know how to get out. When I was 21, I finally had the courage to end it. At first, he was upset, but I was adamant, I was done; then on the day he was supposed to move his things out there was an incident that now seems like another person's life. It resulted in armed police surrounding the house. I used this opportunity, the first time I'd ever seen him scared, to agree I would tell them he would leave without any trouble if he promised to leave me alone and never come back. He did and I could finally breathe for the first time in three years.

After this relationship it sealed what I had always thought – that I would never settle down. I was never the girl that dreamed of getting married and having babies. I liked coming and going as I pleased and answering to no one. A lot of people with ASC struggle with romantic relationships, for many different reasons, some of which I explore in the next section. There is a wonderful TV series on Netflix called 'Love on the Spectrum' which explores this subject, and I recommend everyone to watch it. It brings a lot into perspective, and shows, in varying circumstances, that most autistic people do want to find a life partner, and have a huge amount of love to give, but it can be more difficult for us due to the way in which our brain works. Before my husband, Shaun, I dated a few people and had a couple of boyfriends, but nothing that was serious to me or anything that had a big effect on me. The same as friendships, it takes a lot for me to build on something with someone, and to be honest, I was just happier on my own.

Don't settle for a relationship that won't let you be yourself.

Oprah Winfrey

Television Producer, Author, Actress

RELATIONSHIPS – SECTION TWO

E very single person on this planet is different and has their own issues and personalities so it is impossible to expect us all to have the same relationships. Just like with friendships I think we ALL need to be careful not to compare our relationships with those of other people. Nobody ever knows what goes on behind closed doors so when a couple may seem perfect and too good to be true, that's usually correct. Every couple, and family, must do what works best for them and only the two of you know what that is. I will never explain myself to anyone else and have no desire to do what is 'normal'. Other people's relationships are no business of anyone else except the two people in it, and as nobody is perfect, we should all try to remember not to judge. Of course, if you are asked for advice or input that is a different story.

Unrealistic expectations put a lot of unnecessary pressure on us as individuals and as couples. Do you think other couples: spend more time together? Show their love to each other more? Have sex more frequently? Or argue less than you? Either way it doesn't matter, what should matter is if you are truly happy, if your partner is truly happy and if not, change whatever it is that would make it better, and that might mean to not be together but it's best to be honest with ourselves, and each other. Life is short.

My husband and I have very similar morals and beliefs about family and raising our son and we're both real home birds, we're both more than comfortable to sit together in silence at home or just to go out for a nice meal rather than anything wild, but we are also vastly different. Sometimes this works well, sometimes not so well and that is something we have always worked on and probably always will. My husband is learning what life is like living with someone with diagnosed ASC and ADHD (other than his son) and he is committed to working on our relationship now and in the future, as am I. For example, I often need time alone, to try and gather my racing thoughts and my brain works very differently to his so we do not always see things the same way or have the same opinion, we agree to disagree quite a lot. I personally hate conflict; I take arguments very much to heart and would rather walk away, and talk things through calmly later, than deal with a big row. I also find it easier to communicate difficult things in writing, but he hates to read it. Being autistically black and white, I don't understand how people can have furious fights and then expect to be fine together five minutes later, and the fact that some people seem to love the up and down of fighting and making up is genuinely beyond me. My husband (like many people) can say things he doesn't mean on the rare occasion that he does get angry; however, he will then be over it half an hour later – I react a completely different way. I will remember what has been said, literally for years, and will be unable to return to 'normal' that quickly. I need to give myself time to calm down and think things through logically; minor issues can and do seem huge to me in the moment.

The foundation which we have built over the years has solidified our partnership so we can accept and support each other; we also both know that we're better together, it just works. It does help that our son was diagnosed with ASC aged three, so my husband knew a lot about the condition before I was diagnosed and probably doesn't have the same opinion of it that others without any experience often do. Marriage in general, ND or not, takes work to last a lifetime and I think before people make that commitment, especially when children are involved, we need to really understand this and make sure we choose the right partner (or none). Shaun and I have been together since our early twenties, I am 40 this year, so in that amount of time people do go through changes and grow, so it takes genuine effort to make things work.

Most parents of autistic children struggle in their relationships for many reasons. For example, there can be blame, each parent can have a different opinion to the other about what the condition means for their child and their family, and they can disagree on the ways in which to support their child. Thankfully, no matter what else we might disagree on, Shaun and I are and always have been a team as parents, and both have our own roles to support Jude in the best ways we can. Given the fact that I don't have the capacity to sit and 'play' with toys or the patience to lead someone else who isn't interested into playing a game or completing a learning activity, Shaun takes this side of things and does a great job. My 'job' is managing mostly everything else including arranging and attending all of Jude's appointments, reviews, everything school related, planning and doing all of the school holiday activities and scheduling and preparing for any help that we need, keeping on top of everything that needs to be explained to Jude in advance such as changes in routine/holidays etc, making sure Jude is eating healthily and exercising, organising playdates for him to socialise, planning exactly what activities Shaun needs to be concentrating on with Jude, chasing up (there's a lot of that) and continuously making sure he is getting the best support as he grows and matures and develops more every day – this can be in the form of arranging for new referrals/assessments/reviews (as well as changing things at home when needed) as if we as parents of ND children aren't proactive in doing this it just won't happen. This shouldn't be the case, but it is.

It is believed that around 70% of couples with an autistic child subsequently divorce. It can be highly stressful, especially when the child is young, and unless you have a lot of help, alone time together is almost impossible. Shaun and I spend 90% of our time with our son which can be exhausting, especially for me being ND myself, and we both usually just want to go to sleep when he does. Our son has struggled greatly with sleep for the past couple of years, and one of us has to sleep with him each night or he will NOT sleep at all – at the moment, we're hoping this won't last forever (I detail this further on in 'Parenting A Child With ASC/ADHD'). We rarely have time to socialise together or go out alone, though we do try to have the odd date night and to get away for a couple of nights alone once a year, but for me in particular, the worry about Jude, how he'll cope, the planning it takes to have him looked after and the preparation it takes is huge and can defeat the whole point of taking a break. Jude has never slept out without us past the baby stage – we tried it once a couple of years ago and he slept for just one hour and stayed awake for the rest of the night until 6am. Not only is that unfair to him but also to whoever it is that is looking after him, especially if they have their own children.

Many ND people, due to their sensory issues for one, prefer to have separate bedrooms to their partner which in general is thought of as 'strange' by most people and can cause issues in relationships. I do find that I sleep better when I'm in bed alone, and that's not just with regards to Shaun; I've never been able to sleep well with Jude in the same room either. I hear every little noise, snore, cough, breath, turn in bed etc, there's much less space, and it can be really stressful especially if you struggle with sleep anyway. My bedroom is my sanctuary, my favourite place and it always has been.

Sex for people who are ND can be another minefield which puts a lot of strain on relationships. As mental health issues are higher in those with ASC and/or ADHD, this plays a part, as it does for anyone who suffers with these issues. You're often extremely tired if you suffer with depression and/or anxiety and can lack the energy to engage in sexual activity; it can also be hard to relax enough to be able to enjoy intimacy. In autism, sensory issues can often play a part too, smells, noises, touch, and textures can all be heightened which can mean sex isn't enjoyable and if it's not enjoyable, why do it? Having an understanding partner can help you work through these issues without pressurising you about something that is out of your control. Again, more is being learned all the time but with regards to ADHD a few sex related issues are that females with ADHD can find it hard to orgasm. Many people with ADHD take medication to allow them to manage their lives more easily, but this medication, as with antidepressants, often has an impact on libido. Also, as many people with ADHD have a hyperactive brain, they often cannot relax enough to 'be in the moment'. At the opposite end, there is also hypersexuality where someone with ADHD may have a stronger than average sexual appetite that does not match their partner or even enjoy the thrill of dangerous liaisons which can sometimes lead to promiscuity and poor decision-making.

I'm not sure whether it is 'better' for ND people to exclusively date other ND people, but there really isn't much of a choice anyway regarding who you are attracted to or who you fall in love with. But I do know it's impossible for a NT person to completely understand what life is like for a ND partner and this can and does cause issues. Especially when the ND person themselves doesn't have a diagnosis and are unaware they have a medical condition, they might live constantly telling themselves (and therefore their partners) that things will get 'easier' once a certain phase has passed, for example, when I finish this training course, when I lose this weight, when we have a baby, when we get engaged, when I get the job I want etc, the list can be endless. This is because without knowing the root cause of who you are means you're always waiting to feel like what everyone else seems to feel like, 'normal', but that's not going to happen. There isn't anything wrong with you, you don't need fixing. In turn NT partners can live with the belief that their ND partner is going to change or 'be fixed' which will never happen, and disappointment may set in.

In general, not just related to sex, ND partners will often not have a lot to give at the end of the day. It can be EXHAUSTING to just get through the day with our minds, that when we're home, we just want to be in our comfort zone and do what we need to do to find some peace. NT people can take this as a lack of attention and unkind and unloving behaviour, which they could eventually get bored or resentful of. Also, ND people often don't feel truly 'seen' in relationships. Partners need to get to know us as individuals, what we truly like or don't like, want, or don't want. The ideas that NT people have of happiness or kindness don't necessarily apply to us. For example, for most of us it would be our idea of a nightmare to be surprised with a trip away. That's not ungrateful it's just a difference to NT people. However, if we do find a partner who can support us, who we can communicate honestly with, who loves us for who we are and truly lets us be ourselves, we can be the most loyal, genuine, understanding, and caring people you could meet. It's just about finding the right fit for you – if you even want to; you may be happy as you are, and that's the same for everyone,

ND or not. Again, something we're brought up to believe is that we 'should' meet someone and settle down, but that's not right for everyone.

With that being said, there is a lot to think about and consider, on both sides, of a ND/NT relationship – and neither is wrong, just different. For the ND, are you happy to be never TRULY understood? Will you be willing to repeatedly explain to your partner what it feels like to be ND when they don't seem to acknowledge the difficulties you face? Can you take on the ups and downs of another person and their world as well as your own? And to have to think about someone other than yourself in everything that you do? Will you have the energy to give your partner the attention they need? For the NT, can you honestly accept your ND partner and their condition/s now and in the future? Will you be happy with the fact that they will need to spend potentially a lot of time focusing on themselves? Are you okay with never truly understanding how your partner's mind works/thinks? Will you be okay with the fact that your partner may need to follow strict routines and not be so open to change? Will you be able to feel and show empathy to your partner for their conditions and the difficulties they bring when you don't, and never will truly, 'get it'? Are you willing to learn all you can, now and in the future, about ND so that you can support your partner? Because this is up to you, we shouldn't have to explain our conditions constantly. If it is to be a long term/serious relationship it may be helpful, for both sides, to do some research and honest thinking so that you know what to expect – there are both positive and difficult aspects and of course every person is different.

My husband and I do our best; at times, especially during my own journey through diagnosis etc, it has been unbearably hard for us both, but we believe ultimately, it's worth it. Shaun isn't autistic and he doesn't have ADHD so it's impossible for him to fully understand how I am feeling or just how overwhelmed I can get, and he has off days himself, as he's only human, where it feels like he completely doesn't care or want to care about how I struggle, but we're both learning and growing together in this. We have made an agreement to completely accept each other, warts and all, for who we are as individuals. I do understand that it isn't aways easy being with someone who is ND, BUT I also know that it's not always easy being with anyone for life.

We have both, separately, together and in therapy, spent A LOT of time thinking and discussing what it means for us as a couple being the parents we need and want to be for Jude while he is young. There are days on end where we literally don't get 60 seconds to speak to each other alone, but we have a strong foundation and we both 'get it'. We know it's 'different' and not how we both might have imagined it would be, especially as it greatly differs to our relationship before being parents, but ultimately, we are happy together and we both understand WHY it is this way. I often remind myself that childhood goes so fast and that I should cherish every second – every person who has raised children will tell you this – and I genuinely do. Also working as a team for your child and overcoming so many obstacles together really does make you stronger.

Being completely open in writing this, as I think it will be helpful to other families, I want to share that my marriage has taken a huge amount of work, respect, and love to be what it is. In fact, in the not too distant past, we decided for various reasons that we needed to take time apart. Shaun moved out of our family home for several months and I genuinely had no expectation as to what the outcome would be. At the beginning I was numb and so busy with Jude and normal daily life that I didn't have time to sit and think things through. I needed to let how I felt come naturally over time. We communicated throughout, as of course we were still co-parenting Jude and had to work together to make sure the changes at home didn't affect him negatively. From the start we set rules as to what was/wasn't expected of each other and had a vague timeline that we agreed on as we didn't want an open-ended separation but also wanted enough time to decide on our future as a couple and as individuals.

Shaun went to therapy for his own personal issues and over time we realised that we missed each other. Especially for me as I saw the effort he was making and the positive changes he had made. We also looked at ways in which we could both be happier with life at home. I'm a firm believer in never staying together 'for the children', but this was a big decision for us as we both come from broken homes which has affected us individually in many ways. There was no way that after taking this difficult step I was going to move any way forward unless I was 100% certain that it was the best direction for our, and Jude's, future happiness. Thankfully we both decided that we absolutely wanted to be together and continue with our marriage. It's not and never will be perfect, that was never the aim, but the time apart allowed us both to truly understand what we wanted personally and as a couple. It was the best decision at the time and although difficult was completely worth it to have the positive outcome that we have.

As long as the three of us are happy, then we'll be together.

Happily, ever after is not a fairy tale. It's a choice.

Fawn Weaver

Author and Entrepreneur

OUR NEW LIFE

For very different reasons, Shaun and myself were two lost souls that I believe were meant to find each other and who needed each other. We grew up living two minutes away from each other and he's often said over the years that he wishes we would have got together when we were much younger, but I don't agree because to be the person he needed, and who he fell in love with, I had to experience everything I did first, to become the strong woman that I am. I knew Shaun vaguely because most of my friends had a crush on him when we were teenagers, he was one of those good looking, popular boys who are naturally great at every sport. He is three years younger than me and in high school that's a lot, so I never looked at him that way and as I've mentioned I was a late developer in that area anyway.

In 2010 we met on a night out and, and although I know it sounds clichéd, for the first time someone felt like home, and I had never felt so strongly about anyone. However, he was not perfect, and I had to use all my strength to help us get to a place where we could build what we now have. Shaun was spoiled by his parents and grandparents and did whatever he wanted to do. He had no responsibilities whatsoever, he didn't even have a bank account, and played football for a living which he loved – the total opposite of me. He also loved to drink and gamble, which I now know is quite common in footballers, and is something that he still works on now. We were and still are imperfectly perfect for each other. I'm certain that nobody else would be as good for either of us as we are for each other.

We officially got together in early 2011 and despite how hard it was at times in the beginning (or the first 18 months or so he was a nightmare) I've never wanted anyone or anything else. He would constantly let me down for dates and plans because he'd be drunk or hungover, and he often didn't have any money because he had gambled it all away. Some of my strengths are taking control and problem solving and these have both helped Shaun with his issues – they still do. The reasons I persevered were because I felt for him what I never had before, and I also had a gut instinct that it was meant to be. When he wasn't drinking, I saw the side to him that I knew he could be and wanted to be; nobody else saw that. He absolutely hated himself for upsetting me and letting me down and he hated how drink made him feel, but he was addicted to the whole vicious circle. Shaun's problems with alcohol have been a journey over the years and he eventually decided it's best if he doesn't drink at all. There are different types of problems with alcohol, and I know that most men like a drink and some don't know when to stop, but Shaun was another level. You also can't help someone who doesn't want help, but Shaun did want to change. I was strong enough to support him in doing that. I certainly wasn't a pushover, but I gave him more time and patience than I would have anyone else.

The best thing that happened to us was around three years into our relationship Shaun being signed to a club near London. We're from the Northwest, so we had to relocate miles away from home. He was physically removed from his old drinking haunts and bad influences and had a fresh start. We really enjoyed this adventure and having time literally just the two of us, we really got to know each other and forged our close bond. We had only lived there for several months when I found out I was pregnant. I had never been maternal whatsoever for a long, long time but my biological clock had kicked in when I was around 28 and I really wanted a baby with Shaun. Thankfully we conceived quite quickly, and, like most women, I became a mum the minute I found out I was expecting.

I think generally this is how most mums feel and it takes a while for dads to catch up or even until the baby is born. This is understandable because until that point the dad's life doesn't really change at all, but the mum's does instantly, and it never goes back. I always thought I'd be a hormonal nightmare when I was pregnant, but I was very chilled, Shaun has said it's the most relaxed he's ever seen me. This was because I was content; also because from the day I took that test everything was for my baby. I researched and read everything I could find about what was best for my unborn child and I knew that stress wasn't good so I just tried to be as peaceful as I could, my baby was my new 'hyper focus' (this ND trait is explained in Part Four). I ate all the right foods, drank as much water as I should, took vitamins and generally looked after myself better. We went to antenatal classes, and I did pregnancy Pilates; as I'm a rhesus negative blood type I had to visit the hospital for injections throughout, but other than that it was a healthy pregnancy. Physically I did not like being pregnant, I didn't like how my body looked or felt, I'm used to always being on the go at 100 miles an hour and I had to slow down, which was hard for me.

During pregnancy I was quite isolated because I didn't have any family or friends where we lived, other than a few girls whose partners played with Shaun, and I only saw them at games. As I struggle to really connect to new people, I basically managed the nine months with no other female support, but I was happy in my bubble. I don't think any new parents are prepared for the way in which their life will change before the baby arrives. No matter what people tell you, you just cannot understand until it happens. Also, I think there's a lot not spoken about that really should be, for example everyone talks about the sleepless nights and the dirty nappies, but what about the constant worry? I found this the same for birth, everyone talks about the physical pain and the medical options you have but what about your recovery? Obviously now knowing I'm ND it's more understandable that I was so overwhelmed, and I would never, ever do it again – but would do it a million times over for Jude.

Our most basic instinct is not for survival but for family.

Paul Pearsall

Neuropsychologist and Author

HEY JUDE

On Tuesday 6th May 2014 my life really started, the same day as my son's.

I was 38 weeks pregnant when it was recommended, I be induced. I was as ready as any new mum can be, my bag was packed, and Shaun's football season had just finished so it was as good a time as any. I was told I had something called cholestasis which was a problem with my liver that wasn't good for the baby, so he had to be delivered as soon as possible.

We had found out I was having a boy at 20 weeks as I really wanted to get things organised (obviously); however, I always instinctively knew I would have a boy. I never had any girls' names, and I only ever pictured a boy. We had chosen the name Jude which I loved and still do now, although there are a few more around now than there was then. I was in hospital for three nights before he arrived. They tried a couple of different methods of induction, but it took a while, then when it did happen it happened fast. I started getting mild pain and was told I could get a bath to help then I was taken down to the delivery suite where my waters were broken for me. I then got another bath and within minutes the pain came over me like nothing I had ever experienced or even imagined. I was completely naked and didn't care one bit who saw me. Shaun helped me out of the bath, because I physically couldn't get out myself. I had always planned to have an epidural because a friend of mine had had one and recommended it and I have never been good with pain (autistic people can either have an extremely high pain threshold or be very sensitive to it and I've always been the latter). The midwife covered me up with a gown and I was sat on the bed while the anaesthetist gave me the injection which I didn't feel or even notice at all as I was already in so much pain. Honestly, words cannot describe the pain but the closest I can say is that it felt like every bone in my body was breaking and I was going to die. I know that sounds dramatic but genuinely this is how it felt; it still haunts me now ten years later.

I somehow took total control of myself, I didn't make a sound I just zoned out, shut down and focused on my breathing to calm myself as best I could. Shaun said he was in complete amazement at how I handled this situation – I think most women would agree that men could not do what we do. Once the epidural kicked in things settled but around an hour later when I felt the urge to push, the pressure was horrific. Within minutes an alarm sounded, and a crash team ran in to the room to check on the baby whose heart rate had dropped. Shaun and I were petrified and had no clue what was happening, and this happened another three or four times when the consultant said I would need to go to theatre, and they would try forceps first and if that didn't work, I would need an emergency caesarean. I was rushed down to theatre and given a spinal block which thankfully took every bit of pain away, but I was exhausted and shivering from the anaesthetics. There was a surgeon and a trainee surgeon at my bottom end and as they were using the forceps, although I couldn't feel the pain, I could feel the movement of them banging against my pelvic bones. At that time, I just wanted my baby to arrive safely, and he did.

Jude weighed 7lb 2oz and scored 9 out 10 on the APGAR tests (Appearance, Pulse, Grimace, Activity and Respiration). I had a skin-on-skin cuddle and then he was taken with the midwife and Shaun to the recovery suite while I was (literally) sewn up. I had had an episiotomy and felt like death. It was the middle of the night/early hours of the morning, and I was traumatised; I still am. From the recovery suite I was moved on to the ward with the other new mums and babies and was so grateful to learn the hospital were trialling allowing partners to stay with the mums so thankfully Shaun could stay with us. I couldn't take my eyes off Jude and had always planned to breastfeed; I hadn't even bought any milk or bottles, I was so determined. However, this didn't go to plan. I was in such a bad way that I couldn't sit up in bed at all so couldn't hold Jude properly for him to feed. The midwives were very pushy about breastfeeding and insisted it was fine and I should keep trying; however, I knew something wasn't right and that my baby wasn't getting what he needed. His mouth was so dry, and he had little blisters on his lips, so I got really upset and demanded some milk, which we got, and he guzzled it. The midwives told us they couldn't give away too much milk, so Shaun went out to get some and some bottles and that was how Jude was fed – not how I planned, but as with anything regarding labour and new babies, sometimes you have to just go with it.

After 24 hours in the ward, I couldn't move out of bed and still had a catheter in. The midwives eventually took notice, and a consultant came to see me; he looked at my notes from surgery and said I should have been getting liquid morphine to cope with the pain and I had only had paracetamol – I was then moved to a private room. I managed to get more rest once I had the correct medication and the quiet of a private room, and after a few days I started to feel slightly better. It was depressing after a while being cooped up in hospital with no sunlight or fresh air and I really wanted to get home to my bubble. After a week in total, we were discharged, and I vividly remember wrapping Jude up and carefully putting him in his car seat to finally take him home.

Shaun was a godsend at that time. I had always only wanted Shaun in the hospital with me when I gave birth; my mum and sister and Shaun's mum and nan came to visit us in hospital the day Jude was born and Shaun's dad came the day after, but at home it was just the three of us. I had planned the first few weeks to be like this as I had read how important the first six weeks are in establishing a bond between parents and their new-born. We were in a little baby bubble like every new family; however, my recovery was not easy at all, and Shaun had to make all the bottles and change all of Jude's nappies for the first ten days of his life. This was a man who had no experience at all with babies or children, and it definitely bonded him to Jude and made him the best dad he could possibly be. I had been allowed to take the liquid morphine home with me and was flat out most of the time. After ten days I talked myself into stopping the stronger medication, I had to try and move forward. I continued to take paracetamol, ibuprofen, and codeine for a while longer and was given physiotherapy at the hospital because my coccyx had been bruised by the forceps which was causing my pain, and slowly I started to recover. Six weeks after Jude was born, we drove back home to visit our families and I felt much better, although honestly, I would say it took about a year to feel myself again physically (although I don't think that many women ever feel 100% back to their old selves after having a child). I never put any pressure on myself about my body because I feel like you and your baby's health need to be the priority. It's a miracle what our bodies do, and it is put through a trauma, so needs time to heal.

As I've mentioned, something I was not prepared for, or aware of, is the worry that having a child brought to me. I now know that I feel this more acutely because of my conditions but I also know, from conversations I've had, that most new mums feel this overwhelm. Everyone talks about the pain of labour; more people now know about Post-Partum Depression (which is a good thing) and we're all told that we'll never sleep properly again (true), BUT nobody talks about the constant worry. We do get used to it, we don't have a choice because the worry for your child is there until the day you're no longer on this earth, but it is in my opinion the hardest part of becoming a parent. For example, when Jude was a new-born I would worry constantly about cot death, I had read online about how it was more likely in boys and what ages it affected by percentage. I would tell myself once he got to two-to-three years old, I'd be able to relax more. Then when he started eating solid foods, I was terrified he would choke and then of course along comes his communication issues and obsession with when he would talk. Ultimately, I had to have a word with myself and tell myself I needed to take control of this. I was going to worry away his childhood and when he was 21, think where did it go? I wanted to enjoy his early years because I know they go so fast and you can't get them back, as someone who doesn't believe in regret, I had to choose to make the change. Naturally of course I still worry but I don't obsess, and I do enjoy every single day of being Jude's mum.

When Jude was four months old, I had a fluke fall, that I literally couldn't do again if I tried, and badly broke my wrist. I had to have it reset and have metal pins and a plate put in and I couldn't use my arm for months. I couldn't hold Jude, or feed him or dress him, change his nappy, anything. I was really down about not being able to hold my baby and it was not a good time for me. Both our mums came to stay with us for a few days to help because Shaun obviously had to work but, in the end, we had to get a temporary nanny to be with me and Jude while Shaun was out. I still never left his side, but I was physically useless for him.

Jude was a dream baby and sleeping through by five months old (for a few years at least!). We met up with other mums and their babies from the antenatal class often; I was always very aware that because we didn't live close to family and friends we needed to get out and socialise as much as possible. If there was a baby class, he was in it, baby massage, baby yoga, music group, story time at the library, stay and plays, we did them all. Shaun was at work, so it was me and Jude out and about every day and I loved this time with him. We have such a strong bond, having Jude and being on this journey together has genuinely made me a better person, I know Shaun feels the same, and I am eternally grateful for our boy.

There are places in the heart you don't even know exist until you love a child.

Anne Lamott

Author, Political Activist and Public Speaker

THE JOURNEY BEGINS

When Jude was 12 months old Shaun signed for a new club closer to home and the three of us moved to just over an hour's drive from our family and friends. It was a good time to move, the apartment we had was getting too small and a bit claustrophobic with all of Jude's things and he had started to toddle, so we needed more space. We rented a lovely old house with a big garden and started a new adventure. We loved it there and would have been happy to stay there if we could have moved our families there too. Again, Jude and I joined lots of clubs and Saturdays being match days we would either go and watch Shaun play or go shopping and for afternoon teas; it was a lovely time and again strengthened our family unit.

As Jude grew, I knew there was something a bit different about him: by 18 months he wasn't talking or making any effort to communicate, play with other children or show an interest in anyone other than myself and Shaun. I mentioned this to the health visitor, and she said to give it another few months as some children are a bit slower with milestones than others, but I knew there was something, a mother just knows. Jude was, still is, the most gorgeous boy and that's not just my opinion: everyone who meets him tells me the same. He is also the happiest child and always has been, he very rarely gets upset; I can count on one hand the number of tantrums he's had in his life, he's just an absolute pleasure. I am very grateful that Jude has the ability to stay so calm even when frustrated. I do know that there are many children on the spectrum who struggle more significantly with their behaviours due to severe sensory issues and/or frustration, for example, (which given the difficulties they face is completely understandable!).

I pushed the health visitor, and we got an appointment with a speech therapist, we were then assigned three monthly visits with her, and she gave us advice to follow at home. This wasn't enough in my opinion, but speech and language services are massively overstretched, so we hired a private speech therapist who saw Jude weekly. She told us she thought he had social communication difficulties. It's hard to distinguish anything else when a child is only 18 months old because many things that all babies and toddlers do or behaviours they have, are similar to autistic traits – such as flapping their hands in excitement, playing a certain way with toys and refusing different foods. Due to what I now know is my autistic and ADHD personality I won't let things go if I think more needs to be done and will continue with things until what I know should and can be done, is done. I can be very pushy and thank God because being a parent to a child with additional needs, means you have to fight to get them what they need and deserve.

When Jude was two and a half years old, I had managed to get him on the waiting list for a MDT (Multi-Disciplinary Team) assessment. By this point, I had studied everything I could, day and night, and knew he needed more support. It was a long and difficult process and around the same time we had started planning a move back home and buying a house that we could settle permanently in and prepare Jude for school. Now, as we would be moving to a different county, I was going to have to do the whole process again because once we moved, Jude would be off the list for assessment. However, we travelled a few times to see the additional needs nurses at the child development centre back home and they thankfully agreed to take him on at the position he was at currently. The problem was with speech and language, they didn't take Jude on for 12 months as he had to start at the bottom of their waiting list, despite me calling them weekly. However, by now we had learned so much ourselves that we could communicate with Jude and knew what we had to be doing to help him develop while we waited. Any speech therapist will tell you that the most important work is done at home.

Other than Jude being autistic and therefore his brain working differently, there is no definitive answer as to why he has problems with speech. However, there is a theory, one which I have been told personally by autistic adults who didn't speak until late adolescence, which I believe is justified – that ND children have so much more going on in their minds than those of NT children that at the point of focusing to develop language there are more important things (for them at least) that they are working through and concentrating on that it's just not a priority. Jude is confident, not quiet, not shy and he has a great personality, and I am confident that one day he will speak and be able to share his amazing thoughts, opinions, and ideas with us. However, in the meantime I don't put pressure on him or any of us about how and when this will happen; as I have said, I don't want to wish the time away because it's too precious and I wouldn't change him for the world.

A mother's love for her child is like nothing else in the world. It knows no law, no pity, it dares all things and crushes down remorselessly all that stands in its path.

Agatha Christie

Legendary Author

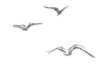

HOME

Another thing that I was dealing with was that since I had had Jude my health issues had not improved. When you have cholestasis in pregnancy it is supposed to go away as soon as you give birth, but my bloods had continued to show inflammation in my liver which I'd never had before. The consultants in both London and our new hospital had been mystified and I had suffered bouts of extreme abdominal pain where I had had to leave Jude safely in his cot while I rolled around the bathroom floor. I'd suffered with what I was told was IBS (Irritable Bowel Syndrome) since I was around 18 years old. It was mostly bloating; I was petite and as soon as I ate anything you could see it in my stomach (this is still the case now and I hate it, especially on holiday). However, once we moved back home, I was referred by my new GP to our local hospital and they arranged a colonoscopy following which I was diagnosed with Crohn's Disease. I was glad I had an answer to my symptoms but anxious that I had a lifelong illness that was unpredictable and could not be healed. I now have check-ups with the consultant twice a year and if I experience any worrying symptoms there is a dedicated team at the hospital who I can contact directly who normally see me the same day. To be fair, touch wood, I suffer mildly compared to some people with Crohn's. If I look after myself, sleep well, eat well and drink well I'm ok and don't get so much pain, although when I do get a flare up it is excruciating and physically stops me doing anything, but I do sometimes feel drained as it is an autoimmune disease. Crohn's disease can affect you literally from the mouth down, not just your bowels, it's also a disease that doesn't make you look ill so people think you're fit and healthy and don't appreciate or understand what it takes out of you, which can be frustrating.

Now at this time, back in our hometown, all moved into our new house, Shaun is commuting each day for training and staying over Friday nights before Saturday's games, it's not ideal for us as a couple, but it is much better being settled for Jude. If it was just the two of us, we could have moved around forever but it wasn't what was best for Jude, especially now he was under the child development team waiting for assessment. I have always envisioned living in a different country, a warm one – I'm not a fan of the UK weather and as time goes on our political issues – but it is home and for this moment in time it is what is best for Jude.

Jude started a local pre-school when he was three years old, and I chose the specific setting he went to as it was attached to a children's centre and a lot of health workers including speech therapists worked from there. I'm so glad he went to this nursery because the staff, in particular the deputy head who was also the SENCO (Special Education Needs Co-Ordinator), were so experienced and helped me above and beyond what I could have expected.

As Jude was non-verbal it was clear he was going to need support in school no matter what his forthcoming diagnosis was or wasn't. The SENCO told me I needed to get Jude assessed as soon as possible so that he could get an EHCP (Education Health Care Plan – this used to be called a Statement of Special Education Needs) because without one there wouldn't be any additional support provided. I obviously had no experience in any of this, but I learned by reading every night until all hours, I was obsessed with getting everything for Jude that he needed, deserved, and was entitled to. I had worked for the council in the past so wasn't intimidated by speaking to them or meeting with them and knew that most of what they will sign off on is dependent on finances. It is a big injustice in my eyes that parents who, for many reasons, cannot, or do not have the ability to do what I managed to do, have children with additional needs that are not supported or even diagnosed, and I would love to help some of these families in the future.

Jude loved pre-school and the staff and other children loved him – that's always been the way and it still is, everyone who meets Jude loves him. Even as he's gotten older and his peers are older, they are still drawn to him, although he doesn't play 'with' them, he likes to be around them. Children can be amazingly understanding and patient, and it's a shame that adults aren't always the same, but I do believe the world is changing and kindness and acceptance will be much more common in future generations.

Jude has five cousins now: one is two years younger; one is three years younger, two are six years younger and one is just six months old. The three little ones are a bit too young to play themselves at the moment, but the two older ones have grown up with Jude and just know, love and accept him for who he is. At different stages they have questioned why he doesn't talk or why he sometimes doesn't seem interested in them (as have a couple of friends' kids of the same age) and I always explain that everyone is different, Jude still loves them and loves being around them (which he really does) and that we all learn things at different times. I give examples they can understand such as, Jude may be able to sleep through the night without a nappy, for example, while one is still not quite there yet, or that Jude can swim without armbands, and one is still learning and that that is absolutely fine.

There are many other methods of communication that Jude has and that he can learn in the future, and in the meantime we all have to understand, that he may need space sometimes and for people to learn to understand him. We spend a lot of time socialising with his cousins, especially my sister and her kids, because I've always wanted him to be around other people, to build relationships and not be wrapped in cotton wool. I also want Jude (and my nieces and nephew) to have a close family unit because I never had that, and I feel it's so important for your entire life. I have a small family, just my mum, sister and brother and us having children has completely changed our dynamic and they have undoubtedly made us closer. As parents we must put the effort in whilst our children are young to make those foundations for them.

Family is not an important thing. It is everything.

Michael J. Fox

Actor and Activist

YOUR SON
HAS AUTISM

Jude had his diagnosis of ASC a few months before he started school. I pushed and pushed the child development team literally every day until we got the assessment appointment with a consultant paediatrician, and it took just 15 minutes. She obviously had all his background info, could see he was non-verbal, his reports from pre-school and whilst in the room Jude was repeating a little routine circuit which she pointed out. Three years old is quite young to receive a diagnosis but because Jude's needs had been spotted early, he was way ahead in terms of the whole process. Most children aren't assessed until they have been to school, and the staff refer them for various reasons, but I knew Jude needed support in place before he started school.

Although I had long suspected Jude may be autistic, the only thing that had ever actually been mentioned to me, by a professional, was social communication difficulties so I still felt shocked for some reason. Any parent who has their child diagnosed will tell you the beginning of the journey is just inexplicably hard. As someone who had no previous knowledge of ASC, it felt like the end of the world. I no longer feel like this, and am really sad that I ever did feel that way because it was totally unnecessary. I am genuinely thankful for who Jude is and would never change anything about him, I now know children with ASC are truly magic and can still achieve whatever they want to. A lot of children with ASC are particularly instinctive about other people, they know if someone is apprehensive of them or unsure of them and they also know someone who is completely open to them without judgement, and they will show you in their behaviour. I have a real affinity with autistic children and see them for who they each are as individuals (more than likely because I understand them) and as a result I am usually treated to lots of affection and attention that only a lucky few experience, and I am so grateful for this. It has changed my life.

Every child, every person, is different. We all have different personalities and quirks regardless of whether we are on the spectrum or not. The abilities that ASC gives to people should be focused on rather than any struggles. For all parents our job is to guide our children, support them, love them, keep them safe and teach them to be happy as themselves. We should always be working on helping them achieve their potential and that is the same for parents with children on the spectrum. I honestly believe that Jude can and will do whatever he wants with his life, whether that's to become prime minister or to work in a supermarket; my only hope for him is that he is happy.

Shaun was, as ever, more laid back than me and told me not to worry and that Jude just is who he is. After lots of discussion we decided, for the time being, not to tell a soul about Jude's diagnosis, except education and health professionals who needed to know. The reason for this was not because we were ashamed (you'd be surprised the number of parents who delay their child getting support because they're in denial about anything 'being wrong' with them and the effect on their 'reputation' when this only prolongs the child's struggles) but because we decided that Jude was three years old, and the only reason we had pushed for a diagnosis is so that he could get the support he needed in school. We didn't want him to be put into a bracket because people don't understand, which often they don't, as well meaning as they may be. We didn't want anyone to treat him any differently; as much as our families loved him, we felt that they would have done so without even realising. Although he was non-verbal (which we told people was still due to social communication difficulties) he didn't display anything else that anyone would point out as 'different'. He didn't have meltdowns, he didn't refuse foods, he wasn't overly bothered by noise or lots of people – this is still the case now. We have always maintained that one of the reasons Jude has these coping skills is because we made sure he was treated the same as any other child by us and everyone else and we still do (albeit sometimes he needs a bit more attention than the average nine year old, and we all need to be more understanding because of his communication difficulties).

I know there are autistic children who have other conditions or disabilities that prevent them from being so exposed to the world, but in general I think it is helpful, for all involved, to take them out into society – to the shops, to restaurants, to fairgrounds, to swimming centres, to soft plays etc and to be around other children and adults from as young an age as possible to get them used to the 'real world'. Jude absolutely loves eating out, going on holiday, going to the fair and theme parks, going swimming and a huge list of other things and we just prepare him suitably – I go into more detail about this in the Advice for Parents section. As much as it may seem kinder to wrap them in cotton wool and let them stay at home all day, in the long run this is no good for anyone, least of all our children because they won't be able to live like this forever, and the more they're used to this the harder it gets to integrate them into society. I also know that sadly there are children and adults that haven't had parents who could do this for them, for many reasons, but I hope that whoever cares for those people now and in the future will be highly trained and genuinely want to support them to reach their potential in life. We can learn and achieve positive change at any age.

All children need is a little help, a little hope, and somebody who believes in them.

Magic Johnson

Retired Basketball Star, Activist and Father

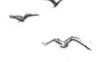

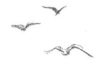

FINDING A
SEN SCHOOL

Now that Jude had his diagnosis, myself and his pre-school set up the final meeting for his EHCP which included reports from an Educational Psychologist, Speech and Language, Occupational Therapy, and many others, plus statements from Shaun and I about how Jude behaved at home and what we wanted him to achieve and what we thought he could achieve. There was no chance Jude was not getting the EHCP, I would have fought anyone I needed to, to get him what he deserved. Thankfully I didn't need to fight any longer as we presented a good case and following a home visit Jude was granted his EHCP, which included funding for full time one-to-one support at school. Now the journey to find a school could begin and it was something I thought long and hard about. We visited a couple of SEN schools and units and a couple of mainstream schools and ultimately decided that at that time the right place to at least start Jude's school journey was at our local mainstream school where I had always thought he would go.

One of the SEN schools in particular was great, and actually allowed me to go back to hear a presentation from a young autistic man who had just graduated from university (which was amazing and the kind of story we ND parents love to hear), but I wanted to at least try Jude being in a mainstream setting. I felt that being around speaking children would help his communication development and social skills, and knew that he would always have his one-to-one with him. I also knew that many mainstream schools nowadays have autistic students, because the capacity to have all autistic children provided with a SEN school is just not possible for many reasons, mostly financial, and not always necessary. I have always been under the opinion that it's best to try and fail than not to have tried at all so that you don't wonder what if, and although mainstream didn't work out for Jude, I am truly glad that we did try.

Jude was in a class of 30 children in an open plan space with a class of another 30 children. He was around 60 children day in day out for a year and a half, and in reception he loved it. He got used to being around other children, he got used to the noise and he did enjoy being around them. He was never sad, upset, or frustrated. He had a wonderful relationship with his one-to-one and I truly trusted her to look after Jude and we had thoroughly discussed how I didn't want him to be held back in any way, which she fully agreed with. He learned how to follow school routine, how to eat lunch with the other children and all the other positive social development that school helps children with. As more and more children are being diagnosed with ASC and ADHD, there obviously is not enough capacity in the current SEN schools we have, so many ND children are recommended to be educated within mainstream schools, which in many cases is very doable; however, this being said, there should be mandatory training for ALL mainstream school staff with regards to these conditions to provide the correct support as it is highly important to the welfare and education of our children.

Soon after Jude started in Year One it was apparent to me that this wasn't going to continue to work moving forward. The big change that ALL children feel in that transition was magnified for Jude – he didn't have the ability yet to be able to sit at a desk and do the 'work' set, he needed to be able to move around the classroom and get some exercise and have downtime. He needed sensory stimulation and quiet time/breaks. As good as the school was, and we did have a great relationship with all involved, they just didn't have the facilities to meet his needs; although they said there was always a place for him, and they would do their best, I knew it wasn't best for Jude. I'm not an overly emotional person but I was honestly heartbroken that he had to leave; nevertheless, it wasn't about me, and I know now that him leaving is the best decision we could have made. Little did I know how hard it would be to get to that point, however.

The road to finding a SEN school for your child is an extremely hard one. In all the training courses I have attended over the years, ND courses, communication courses, device courses, the list is long, and all the amazing families whom I have met along the way (all at different stages of their child's journey), this is always a huge obstacle. A big issue is finances – local authorities don't have the number of SEN schools that are needed and to send children to a private or out of town school costs a lot more than they want to pay. Of course, I do know their budgets and funding are ultimately set by the government, but either way it isn't good enough. You shouldn't have to battle like I did to get your child into a school that is suitable for their needs. If all children with additional needs were educated in a place where staff are trained well for their conditions, the difference to their whole lives and society would be huge.

As is usually the case, I took the matter into my own hands, because I will never wait around for anyone else to decide on my child's future when time is short. Once we had spoken to Jude's school a meeting was called with the local authority (they monitor EHCPs) and it was agreed that Jude was suitable for a place in a SEN school, but that the problem was going to be finding one. In our county there are currently only two SEN schools, one of which is for children with more physical disabilities and one which is mainly for children with ASC. This school is over-capacity and has a huge waiting list (this is the one I went to the presentation at when Jude left pre-school). I knew I would have to look out of town, so I researched all SEN schools in the wider area and contacted them; several were over-capacity, and some didn't have a class that would be suitable for Jude due to age. I visited a few that could possibly take him, but to me they were not suitable for Jude. Like any school, you know as soon as you visit, and speak to the staff and the children, see the whole setting, if your child will fit in and flourish there. One of the schools' staff mentioned to me that there was a brand-new school in Liverpool (we live on the outskirts) for children with ASC and I immediately looked it up. School B is an independent school and had been purpose-built for children on the spectrum; amongst other things they have a hydrotherapy pool, trampoline room, soft playroom, sensory room, no bright colours – everything kept neutral so as not to overstimulate, and the reviews from the parents who had children there already (it had been open 12 months) were great. So, I called and arranged a visit with the Head and was shown around this wonderful school that was the only place I could see my son. When she took me in to the pool area, I become very emotional (not like me at all but Jude's absolute favourite thing is swimming) and I knew Jude needed a place there. Even better was the room they have fitted out as an apartment where the children learn life skills such as cooking and cleaning (all these things should be taught in ALL schools in my opinion, but that's another story). The problem was there was only one place left, a few places were held for children who had ongoing circumstances to be resolved, and many things weren't on my side, the main one being the school was not under our local authority.

As I drove home, I called Shaun and said this was THE school and he trusted me although he hadn't seen it – I have always taken care of this side of things because it's what I'm good at (hyperfocus can be a superpower of ASC and ADHD) and he works full-time. I then called our local authority and told them I had finally found the school and asked them what needed to be done to move forward, emphasising that there was only one place left. I then called the head office of School B and told them we desperately wanted the last place for Jude but that we were at the liberty of our local authority. I must have driven the intake officer mad in the weeks and months whilst we were waiting for confirmation from our local authority, but he was great – I have found it's often the case that people who work in SEN settings are generally more helpful and understanding than those in mainstream. The local authority said they had never heard of this school so would need to look into it first. I sent them all of the information from the school and chased them up every day either by email or phone or both. Someone from the SEN department eventually went out and visited the school, as they must see if they think it is indeed suitable for the child in question. This took weeks to arrange and then it was taken to a panel which is held once or twice a week to make decisions on different children's needs. On the day of the panel, I called later in the afternoon to get an update and was told that they wouldn't be happy to fund a place there for Jude as it was too expensive, it was more than double that of a place in a state SEN school.

Now, whilst I completely understand that the government don't have an unlimited amount of money, I also know that they throw all kinds of money into areas that are not of high importance, whereas education is one of, if not the most, important area we have in society. Money was not going to be the reason why my son didn't go to a school that would best support him, so not being experienced in such matters we offered to pay an amount of money ourselves if the local authority could just budge a bit higher on their end. I was told this had never been asked before so again it had to go back to panel, and panel decided it wasn't 'appropriate' for us to do this. I was told they would continue looking into schools themselves, but I advised them I had looked at every SEN school in a 20-mile radius and this was the only one that was available and suitable. I must add that these 'panels' were often cancelled or delayed due to staff shortages so decisions always took much longer than they should have. Remember this is just one child so the number of children that are being under-served blows my mind and it is something else I would love to help change in the future; it should not be so difficult for our families. Again, I do want to point out that many of the staff that work within the SEN departments within local authorities are usually extremely overworked and as much as they do care for these children and want to help, they are ultimately very limited by 'the powers that be'.

The next day I contacted the Education Rights Service, who I had seen advertised by another family on the social media page for the National Autistic Society, and they were super helpful and supportive and told me they would pass my details on to the Tribunal Service because that is the route we would have to take at this point. The very next day I got a call from the Tribunal Service, again so supportive, they told us that no amount of money should be the deciding factor in giving a child, who it had been agreed needed it, a place at a SEN school. They also told me I should never have offered a penny towards the fees (so now I know but at the time we were just desperate and would literally have done anything to get Jude there). After this conversation, I called the local authority and updated them that we would be taking this matter to tribunal and the change was instant. Our local authority's SEN department was already under scrutiny due to poor performance, so they absolutely did not want this to go down that route. I was told that they hadn't said a definite no to School B (they had) but that they needed time to look themselves. The Tribunal Service said they had 14 days to do this, and I had to wait exactly 14 days until they came back to me and finally agreed that there wasn't anywhere else suitable for Jude in the wider area. I understand procedures must be followed but the time that was being wasted was not beneficial to anyone, least of all Jude. School B was then taken back to panel with the local authority and then the first 2020 pandemic lockdown hit.

Most council staff were now working from home, and panel scheduling had been thrown up in the air, so there were more delays, but once they did finally manage to have a Zoom panel meeting the school was agreed for Jude; however, the costings needed to be signed off by the finance manager before we could get our hopes up. I spoke again with the Tribunal Service, and I believe they sent an email into the SEN team to try and help our case. I was told the finance manager would be back in the office the next day, so I called later the next afternoon for an update and was told they couldn't reach her. At this point I lost my composure; I had gotten to know all the staff and the department manager by name (I'm sure they dreaded me calling) and I was crying and telling her this whole thing was making me physically ill. It had been five months or more since we started and it was getting beyond difficult, Jude had been stuck in a school, who whilst they cared for him, wasn't right for his needs and I couldn't think of anything else but the pressure on my shoulders day and night of getting this right for him. It was a Friday afternoon so I knew the offices would now be closed for the weekend and I was just at a loss of how long I could keep hearing the same apologies and promises. However, ten minutes later the manager called me back and said it had all been agreed, Jude could take the place at School B.

By the Monday afternoon the Head had called me asking when Jude would like to start – Jude's mainstream school had closed a couple of weeks previously due to the lockdown but as this was a SEN school that wasn't compulsory, and he started on the Wednesday. We had been cautiously preparing him for a new school over the weeks beforehand, and the fact he hadn't been in school for a couple of weeks also helped the transition, and obviously the wonderful SEN staff who know exactly how to manage children with ASC were amazing.

As time goes on and Jude grows, his needs may change but he is very settled into this school with the most amazing resources, and whatever happens, we'll make sure Jude gets the education and support that he deserves to continue his progress and development for the future.

Everybody is a genius, but if you judge a fish by its ability to climb a tree, it will live its whole life thinking it is stupid.

Albert Einstein

Historical Theoretical Physicist

Part Two

Mental Health

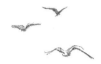

MENTAL HEALTH
– SECTION ONE

Trigger warning – The following chapters may trigger people who struggle with their mental health.

This information may be helpful for those who have loved ones who suffer and want to understand, or for anyone that wants to learn about the subject.

For those who feel like they struggle with their mental health no matter what they do, this information could help you look at other conditions that may have been completely undiagnosed – meaning all generic treatment methods of medication/therapy etc will not be beneficial for you, because your true issue isn't being treated. This was the case for me, and I believe many, many people, particularly females, are the same.

Jude being diagnosed I would say was the first sign for me that I was struggling mentally. The constant worry about his future sent my anxiety into overdrive and I'd never experienced anything like it, I felt like I was losing my mind. I have always been an overthinker and very disciplined in my ways and that was just me, we all have our ways, but this was another level. One of the training courses Shaun and I went on, with some other parents, had a topic 'what the world would be like if everyone was autistic' and I identified with practically every trait listed; it highlighted things like, everyone would be open and honest and it wouldn't be perceived as rude, and people would say what they mean instead of having hidden agendas or dropping hints. I said to Shaun "that's me, that's my world!". Although looking back now I have always been different, I've always liked routine and been super organised, I've always liked being in control, and as I've detailed struggled making friends, BUT I've also always been physically fit and healthy and mentally strong. But now I could feel myself unravelling, it was like a clock was ticking and I knew it was going to explode at some point, I knew I couldn't possibly continue living like this.

Shaun and I got married in 2018 and I spent the year before planning, which I always thought I would love, and I think I would have if we had married before we were parents, but given the little free time I now had, it was like a chore on top of everything else I had to do, and it added to my stress levels. We got married in Cyprus and only wanted a small, intimate wedding, but still I found the organising completely overwhelming. Our wedding day was genuinely the best day of my life, everything went to plan, and Jude had a great time which had been a big worry for me, that, and who would look after him so we could enjoy our day (I really struggle with other people looking after Jude which I detail more in My Journey). I truly enjoyed every moment and let my hair down. We all have the best memories of it.

Just before our wedding, I seriously hit a wall with my mental health and spoke to my friend on the phone about how I was feeling (something I never do) and accepted that I needed to get some help. I sat Shaun down and told him how overwhelmed I was; this wasn't easy because I'd always been in control, I liked to appear to have everything together, but I was drowning. Unless you yourself have suffered with mental health issues you can never understand how it feels, and Shaun is a naturally happy, laid-back person who has never suffered (which I am so thankful for). He listened and took in what I had said and agreed that I needed some help. Speaking about things helped a lot (the saying "a problem shared is a problem halved" is very true) and with the wedding coming up I didn't want to start the whole process with my GP, with possibly medication involved, to affect that time, so I planned to make an appointment as soon as we were home. Around this time, I was also in consultation with the hospital regarding the possibility of starting medication for my Crohn's or even having surgery to remove the affected part of my bowel, but again I refused to go into anything further until after the wedding.

As well as everything else, when Jude started school, I had begun a small clothing business from home. It's something I had always wanted to do. I really enjoyed it and it gave me something for me other than just being a mum and a wife, which I think is important. However, I put that much time and effort in (literally some days staying awake working the whole night through) that it took off in a big way, much more successfully than I had ever planned or hoped for, and it started taking over my life. I was Mum during the day and then working all night, and that time-bomb ticking on my mental health got louder.

After the wedding I started medication and Cognitive Behavioural Therapy to help with what my GP said was anxiety. Once I reached the maximum dose of the first medication I had been put on, I felt it helped slightly, so I stuck with that and hoped for the best and I enjoyed going to therapy. I had never really spoken about my feelings or past or anything personal, I seem to always ask people about their lives, so this was good for me. We spoke about my childhood and Jude, and I told her how after everything I'd learned about ASC, I thought it was possible that I was also autistic, and she agreed. She referred me to be assessed and that was the start of my ND journey – however, the assessment took over a year to come through. I am so grateful to this therapist for referring me because so many people go undiagnosed and live in torture.

In 2020 the pandemic arrived and like most people I found it hard, being autistic not knowing the end game is extremely difficult (although at this point of course I didn't have my diagnosis yet). But I've always needed a plan, I need to know what's happening and obviously during those times nobody did, and although I tried my best, towards the end of 2021 I hit my lowest point so far. The business I had worked so hard on suffered greatly, as many small businesses sadly did. I retreated into myself more and more, even at home, and just wanted to be alone with my constant thoughts. I specifically remember breaking down in tears to Shaun, and being forced to open up again about just how I bad I was really feeling. It was harder somehow now because I had naively thought that because I'd had therapy and was on medication, the issue was resolved and life could go on, but it wasn't, and it couldn't continue how it was. It's very hard to try to explain to someone who hasn't suffered with their own mental health how it feels, especially for me, someone who has always prided themselves on being strong and independent. It sounds stupid now, but I didn't want my husband to think I wasn't perfect; of course I'm not and neither is he, nobody is, but when you're suffering with your mental health you don't think logically. I'm not an emotional person and very rarely cry, but I was sobbing and just so sad that I was still going through this. When you're stuck in that cycle it feels never-ending. I also hated that I had to put worry onto my husband's shoulders, but marriage is a partnership and neither one of you should suffer alone, you're there to support each other and I'm thankful I have that. From then on, I have been very transparent with Shaun about how I'm feeling, and mental health is an open topic in our house.

There is still, in 2024, a huge stigma around mental health. It's ingrained into our society and will take many years to completely change, but the fact is that people die because of this stigma.

I know older generations were raised to 'toughen up' or 'suck it up' or 'life is hard you just have to get through it' but that, A, was in a different world altogether to the one we're living in and, B, an outdated notion that helps nobody. Also, as knowledge and treatments have improved over the years we don't have "to just get on with it". For example, an older lady I know recently told me how she was getting sick of people talking about menopause on television. She said that in her day "we just had a nervous breakdown and carried on". Obviously to me I thought but why should we do that now if there are options that can make things easier? Outdated opinions also stigmatize medication or therapy as far-fetched or that people who need to use these aids as weak – this needs to stop. The brain is an organ, and like every other organ in our body it can get sick or need help. Nobody would think someone with a heart problem was weak for taking medication to help it work better. It's that simple and blows my mind that anyone thinks otherwise.

Unless you have suffered with your mental health personally, you cannot begin to imagine how difficult it is; in my opinion it's worse than being physically sick because more likely than not in that case you can take a tablet or have a lie down and feel at least slightly better, but that's not possible when you're battling with your own mind. It is genuinely painful to not be able to enjoy the life going on around you, and for no reason that you can explain. There is absolutely NO SHAME in getting help or speaking to a therapist for ANYTHING you're struggling with; in fact, it takes more strength to ask for help than to not – a common misconception is that people who struggle with their mental health are weak; in fact they are the strongest people you will ever know, because to survive the agony of your own mind torturing you takes more than those lucky enough not to suffer, will ever understand. Many other countries around the world use therapy like we use dentists, but in our society it's still thought of by most as 'crazy' or 'soft' but that's simply untrue, especially if you have children and you want to improve your mental health to enjoy a better quality of life with them. I openly speak to anyone about my mental health now and will answer any questions about what I have experienced, I will tell people that I take medication and have had therapy. The reason for this is not for attention or because I like to overshare (I'm the exact opposite), but because if even one person hears me and it makes them feel better about doing that for themselves, or a loved one, then it's worth it.

Statistics say that 50% of us will struggle with our mental health at some point in our lives, but I think that number is much higher, especially in today's world where there is the constant narrative every single day that we should look a certain way or live a perfect life, especially for women – which actually, NOBODY in the world does. NOBODY is above having mental health issues, and NOBODY is above being ND or having a ND child – that's just a fact. Social media in my opinion is both a blessing and a curse, it's a great free marketing tool for businesses which I myself have benefited from and it's great for sharing helpful knowledge, but I don't have any personal social media because it's, one, not good for my mental health to see such rubbish and, two, I don't buy in to sharing my life to make it look perfect and possibly making other people feel like they're not good enough. We ALL have ups and downs in our life, that is a fact, life isn't meant to be a bed of roses, that's what makes it so eventful. It is true that going through hard times and conquering them makes the good times better – if things were always perfect how would anything excite us or make us feel happy? How could we appreciate the ups without the downs? I really do try to find the lessons in everything that tests me – I feel like overcoming things makes us who we are.

Our mental health and wellbeing must be our priority, every day, for ourselves and for future generations. It is absolutely true, that you can't care for others unless you care for yourself first. There are many ways in which we can improve our mental health whether you think you suffer or not, it's good to keep our brains healthy, as much we do the rest of our bodies – I provide more advice regarding this in the section 'Helpful Tips'. Now, alcohol is something that I'm not a big fan of, especially with regards to mental health. For the people that can genuinely drink in moderation, like everything else I suppose that's fine; however, I know that many people drink much more than they should, and this really doesn't help either physical or mental health. I think as a society, which I do think is changing in the younger generations, drinking is ingrained into us as fun, normal, and acceptable when it shouldn't be, as it benefits nobody but the people that sell it. As I have mentioned, many ND people drink to numb the chaos in their mind; however, this is only a temporary solution, the same as for people with mental health issues, and we really need to actively try and reduce this. It's a vicious circle because the more you drink, ultimately the worse you feel, in every way, but it's a very much available and promoted substance so it's a difficult cycle to break.

If we could look in to each other's heart and understand the unique challenges each of us faces, i think we would treat each other much more gently, with more love, patience, tolerance and care.

Marvin J Ashton

Influential Author

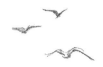

MENTAL HEALTH
– SECTION TWO

At the end of 2021, we were in the middle of a worldwide health pandemic, and I couldn't see my GP face-to-face, so all subsequent contact had to be over the phone. The way in which people with mental health issues are treated is another real problem that I have understanding, and I think anyone who has experience with this knows it needs to change but as with most things it's about funding. My GP and I decided that I should try another medication, so I had to carefully taper off the one that I had been taking for almost two years, and slowly build up on a new one – which didn't have any effect at all. I tried another one which in the first week made me physically sick so that was stopped, and I had a few weeks where I tried nothing at all (all under the guidance of my GP which should always be the case); at first, it seemed fine, but I had a dramatic downturn after around three weeks and was the worst I had ever felt up to that point. I vividly remember one Saturday evening being sat at the kitchen table with my son while he ate his dinner just waiting for my husband to get home from work so I could sit in a quiet room to try and calm my mind which had just been racing all day, I was literally counting the seconds in my head (all whilst trying to appear 'normal' to Jude). I genuinely thought I can't do this anymore, "I think I need to take myself to hospital to be looked after" because I felt so bad, but I finally went to sleep and felt slightly better the next day and called the doctors' surgery urgently on Monday morning.

There are several popular quotes that tell you things like, "keep going – tomorrow will be better", "it's a bad day not a bad life", "it's ok not to be ok" and that "it will pass". This is all true and I tell my son often, so that he can understand his feelings, that we all have different feelings, that nobody is happy all day every day, but not to worry as we will always be happy again soon. I don't believe in sharing much of the adult world with children but I do know that lots of kids suffer in silence so it can only be helpful to talk to them about their emotions and feelings. Also, having a ND child, whose little mind I know is constantly thinking, I think it's even more important to highlight this.

The process of trialling medication is a hard and lonely one because you sometimes feel like nothing is going to help or you get your hopes up about a new one just for it to not work for you. All I can say is, be as strong as you can, allow it time, be open with your friends and family or if you don't have any there are many online forums you can chat on where many people have been through the same process or helplines you can call such as the Samaritans. Believe that things will get better but that this is a part of your journey, and nobody's journey is perfect no matter how much it looks like it. Maybe take a break from social media, rest as much as you need to, but don't lie in bed all day no matter how much you feel like it. Get up, have a shower, get dressed even if it's just fresh pyjamas, and do something that makes you feel good even if it's watching a favourite TV programme or film, keeping a routine is very important. You will get to know yourself and your mental health very well, you will also discover that there isn't a cure, mental health challenges will most likely always be a part of your life, but it doesn't have to ruin your life if you find ways to get through the hard days.

This time was a real eye opener for me, I finally understood and still do, how people can take their own lives. In the past I had always thought it was a selfish act especially when parents do it because how could they leave such sadness behind for their children? However, the fact is that there are different scales and types of mental illness and when someone is suffering so badly, and usually have been for a very long time, they do not think at all except how much pain they are in, and some genuinely believe that their families and friends will be better off without them. These people are victims of their illness and cannot see a way to live their life living in such pain or struggling so hard every single day. Even if you have good days or long periods of not struggling, those bad days can override everything and remind you they're still there and always will be, and it can feel hard to imagine carrying on. I have never felt suicidal, but at times I have thought "how can I possibly live like this for another 50 plus years? I don't want to, it's too hard", but Jude is my saviour. A therapist once told me that although becoming a mother has been hard at times, Jude is my magic and I loved that, and he really is.

There have been many days I've not wanted to get out of bed but have talked to myself in my head to just keep going step by step and sometimes that's all we can do, especially when you have children and no other option, you must keep going. It is a scary thought that our brains can make us believe and do things that we wouldn't do if we were thinking rationally, and again, this is why I am so open with my husband about how I'm feeling and also so that he is able to spot if I am anywhere near that headspace. I cannot say enough how important it is to be aware of your own thoughts and feelings. Be honest with yourself, if you regularly struggle with feeling low or unhappy or overwhelmed, please ask for help. NOBODY ELSE CAN

DO THIS FOR YOU. NOBODY ELSE TRULY KNOWS HOW YOU THINK AND FEEL. Make an appointment with your GP and be completely honest – only then can you start the journey to feeling better. There isn't one treatment that fits everyone, but if you persevere and keep going you can and will live a better life.

For those that feel truly unable to carry on, please take yourself to hospital, there are specialists and facilities who treat those at the very lowest end of the mental health spectrum. I know that on the hard days it feels like there is no point in carrying on, it feels too much, it feels never ending and we can forget the positives in our life or the opportunities that are out there; however, please just tell yourself that it is your mental health making you feel that way. Your life is not hopeless, there is support, there are treatments, and you can feel good enough on more days than not, to see you through the hard days. You just have to ask for help, stay strong, keep going and learn to understand yourself. Life is worth it – you must make your life, in between the bad days, worth it, by being yourself, being honest and making your life what you truly want it to be. In the UK, our NHS currently doesn't have the best reputation with regards to GPs; however, in my experience it's much the same as staff who work in education or children's services. Most GPs do want to help but they are limited by the targets, funding, and other obstacles that they are given. If you don't feel that your GP is listening to you or helping you or that you just don't 'fit', ask to see another GP who may be more helpful and understanding; with regards to mental health and ND this really is crucial because you don't want to have to keep repeating yourself to different doctors. You need someone who understands your history and who you have a bond with. The GP I have had for the last few years is great, which genuinely makes such a big difference and although she can't be available as much as I would like that isn't through fault of her own.

I want to point out that I am also aware that mental health has become a bit of a 'buzz word' for some people, along with the growing awareness and tide of change, there are some people who flippantly use the words anxiety or depression or say they're depressed or anxious if they're having a bad day or week. There will always be people who take advantage of things in this way or who are just ignorant to those that genuinely suffer, and sadly it dilutes the real epidemic that our country has with mental health because it can make it seem less important than it is if everyone is throwing these words around. Those who are genuinely suffering, need support and understanding, not eye rolling or judgement. Yes, every person on the planet has bad days or will feel sad at times, if they suffer a bereavement or have a relationship breakdown etc, but the difference is that this will be for a relatively short period of time and is manageable. They won't genuinely be thinking that their life is too hard to continue living.

Also, most importantly, people with mental health issues will struggle if their life is 'perfect', there doesn't have to be a reason. You can have all the money in the world, a great relationship, enjoy your work, be physically healthy and have lots of friends BUT if you have a mental health condition none of that will help because unless you're treating the imbalance within your brain, in whichever way is best for you, the cycle will continue.

A loud reminder to always check in on your friends and family as often as you can just so they know that you're there and that you care. Particularly the strong ones who you don't think would ever need to know this because, take it from my experience, it is those people who need it the most. Also please don't tell anyone struggling with anxiety or depression to 'snap out of it' – this isn't possible. We are aware that we may be being difficult or are hard to be around, but we CANNOT help it, it's not a choice we have made. Believe me, it's harder for us and small acts of kindness and understanding have a big positive effect.

Everyone you meet is fighting a battle you know nothing about.

Robin Williams

Legendary Actor who died by suicide in 2014

Part Three

Being Diagnosed

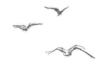

DIAGNOSIS ONE

It took just over a year for a date for my ASC assessment to come through, but once I was finally at the top of the list, things moved quite quickly. I was sent some questionnaires to complete and given some information about what the assessment would entail. It was a quite an intense four-hour interview and included discussing everything you can think of right back from when I was born. If possible, it is encouraged to take along someone who knew you as a young child, but I didn't feel comfortable having my mum there, so I was asked to provide school reports which, luckily, I have. They also called my husband privately to ask him some questions about me and our relationship etc – we've been together for 13 years and have lived together for 12, so he knows me better than anyone else. It was a bit like therapy so not uncomfortable, but it was just a lot to do in one session (I was given a break). However, by this point I was very keen to get things moving either way (diagnosis or no diagnosis), so I was happy to just finally be getting somewhere. I was told all the information that had been collected needed to be taken to a panel of different health specialists the next day and then hopefully an answer could be given.

It was two or three days later that I returned to the clinic and was told that I did have ASC. To be honest, the longer I had waited for this assessment over the last year, the more I knew in my own mind that I was autistic, but it was good to have it officially confirmed, to finally have some answers about why I was how I was, why I had always felt different. I was given a lengthy report and some information to look at, regarding support available and information for family and friends. On the way home, I called Shaun and my sister, both of whom already knew the result as I did. The few friends that I had told, about my journey, were happy for me that I now had actual confirmation, but again had known what the outcome would be.

One thing I did ask when I got this diagnosis, was why have I found being autistic harder to manage as I've gotten older? If you have ASC you're born with it, it's not something that develops later in life or traits that you pick up. I was told that although ASC doesn't worsen as you get older (in many ways it gets easier to manage, for example many autistic children find it easier to live with as time goes on because of experience), high amounts of stress or trauma can trigger your autistic traits to present themselves more than what they have in the past, you quite simply cannot continue to mask for the rest of your life, particularly when you have other difficulties to deal with. Of course, when we have children and other adult responsibilities and stresses, our ND becomes harder to manage. Also, in women our hormones play a big part in the difficulties we face, it is hard being a woman in general, especially at the time of the month, but PMT (Pre-Menstrual Tension) can highly affect those of us who are ND. Our hormones fluctuate throughout the month, throughout our whole lives in fact. Many women with ADHD struggle more when they become perimenopausal and this can be very difficult until after menopause. I detail this more in the section 'Neurodivergent Women'. Not every month but most, the days leading up to my period can be hell, but at the very least now I know why and can explain to myself the logic behind why I am feeling so low, agitated, impatient, unable to concentrate and unpredictable, and that it will pass.

As yet there isn't a medication that can make life easier for autistic people and their specific difficulties; however, many people with ASC do suffer with some form of mental health issues in their life – particularly anxiety – which there is lots of treatments available. There are medications that can help people manage symptoms of ADHD which I will explore in the next section. I will also detail the things I have learned, over time, that help me and my son in our daily lives. I also want to point out that the world does NOT need a cure for ASC. Even the thought of that disgusts me and the fact that there are people, and supposed 'charities', out there looking into this is beyond belief – there are also camps and programmes in the United Sates for one where they pledge to reverse someone's ASC – this is not possible, and neither should it be nor why would any parent want to put their child through this?! Similar to the disgusting camps that claim to 'cure homosexuality' – it is impossible!

As I've explained, ND is just a difference. There are positives and negatives about being ND as there are for any human being. Some of the most intelligent and successful people in the world, who have made ground-breaking inventions that we use every day, are on the spectrum or have ADHD (I have listed some at the end of Part Five). The world needs ND brains like every other kind of brain. Instead of wasting money trying to reverse biology, what should be done is using that money to help support autistic people and their families, to research and to publicise awareness, knowledge, and acceptance.

Once I had my ASC diagnosis, it helped me understand and accept myself better and I know it helped others around me understand me slightly better too (although not everyone has a lot of knowledge about the spectrum and again it's hard to really understand when you haven't experienced it yourself).

After a few months I wasn't feeling a great deal better on the new anxiety medication from my GP and again returned to therapy to try and work my way through what I was feeling. I chose a therapist who had a lot of experience with ND and in my first session she asked me if ADHD had been mentioned at my ASC assessment. I said it hadn't and that the clinic I had been seen at was solely an ASC unit. I had absolutely no knowledge of ADHD at this point, I wasn't even aware that the two conditions could coexist because they contradict one another quite a lot. I now know that people with ASC are highly likely to also have ADHD. More is being learned all the time about the two conditions being linked and currently around 50% (if not more) of people known to have ASC will also have ADHD. I look forward to future research teaching us more about this connection and further support being available. I, probably like most people, imagined it was just children who were diagnosed with ADHD. Except when I was a child full of energy, I have always been the opposite of physically hyperactive, I love my sleep and hate exercise. However, as I came to learn this was all just lack of information and/or generalisation that we pick up from the world around us.

You can't change who you are, and you shouldn't be asked to.

Jonathan Mooney

Author

DIAGNOSIS TWO

I now had something else to learn about, ADHD, and the more I did the more I realised it was also a part of me, and like ASC, it always had been. Now well into this journey of self-discovery (I know this sounds very clichéd but there really isn't another description I can use) I was on a mission and wasn't happy to wait another 12 months-plus to get a diagnosis. I discussed it with my GP, and she did refer me to the NHS ADHD assessment team for their waiting list following an initial written assessment; however, as I luckily had the means to see someone privately, I researched clinics in the local area and found a psychiatriatic clinic who could see me much sooner. It was a detailed process again, as in there were a lot of questionnaires and discussions with the health team before I could be accepted for a full assessment, but after they had all my information, background and reports they agreed I was applicable. I visited Dr N, a psychiatrist who also works in an NHS mental health unit, and we had a conversation for around 90 minutes (before which he had already reviewed all my history etc) and he diagnosed me with ADHD. He noted that there were no other mental health conditions that would explain my issues, such as bipolar disorder, schizophrenia, or personality disorder. I simply had been living my whole life with undiagnosed ASC and ADHD.

There have been many reports in the media recently about private clinics giving ADHD diagnoses. Apparently, there are even social influencers recommending clinics they have collaborated with as it has become 'popular' to have this condition. Firstly, if you do get a diagnosis from a private clinic, unless you can continue to pay for reviews and prescriptions (which the majority of people cannot) you will eventually need/want your care to be transferred over to the NHS. However, when this happens the NHS ADHD Team will have to reassess you and as many private clinics are not following the correct diagnosis process, if you in fact do not have ADHD, they will not provide treatment or accept the diagnosis. This is just one of the reasons for the current huge waiting lists.

As with mental health, there are always going to be people who take advantage or don't take things seriously, not thinking about the people who genuinely struggle. Again, this just causes more problems for those of us who want our conditions, or those of our children/loved ones, to be taken seriously as people get sick of hearing about the 'new trend' which belittles the reality of it. There really isn't a lot we can do about this except try and ignore it, but I would urge anyone who is fed up with reading about this subject to remember that there are people with this VERY real condition – that is medically proven. I've even read that some think that people are keen to get a diagnosis so they can get ADHD medication which are sometimes stimulants. However, the stimulants that are used to treat ADHD will only work if a person has that chemical imbalance in their brain that needs treatment. If not, they have no effect. Also, the majority of people who seek help from private clinics are doing so because they desperately need help and the NHS waiting times for assessments are currently four years long or more in many areas. A GP cannot diagnose ASC or ADHD, nor can they prescribe ADHD medications, so if someone needs that treatment to stop themselves from genuinely feeling suicidal then they shouldn't be berated for it.

PLEASE, IF YOU DON'T KNOW ENOUGH ABOUT THE SUBJECT, DON'T JOIN THE BANDWAGONS OF DOUBTERS.

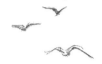

MEDICATION

Thankfully (in my opinion) there are medications that can help people with ADHD manage the difficulties it can create in their lives. Before this whole process, I didn't take any medication for anything, I rarely even took paracetamol, and I had even stopped taking the contraceptive pill after having my son because after not using it for a year, I just didn't want chemicals in my body that weren't naturally there. However, I have had to accept that, for me, medication is needed to enable a better quality of life. As I was to learn, however, it would be another case of trial and error to find the right one for me. There are fewer ADHD medications than there are for anxiety and depression, but two in particular have a high rate of success. As every person's body chemistry is different there is no one-fits-all medication and, as yet, there isn't a guaranteed test to tell you what the best medication for you is (although it is being worked on which will make things much easier for everyone). Frustratingly, we have to trial some different medications and dosages but, in my opinion, it is worth it when you do find the one that works for you because it can genuinely be life changing.

After I started on the first ADHD medication, I had no side effects at all but there was also no benefit from it, although I did try three different doses. This process lasted around two months as you need to give it time to feel any changes (although ADHD medications do work significantly quicker than antidepressants which can take several weeks to even feel a slight benefit and can be difficult to stop taking). Luckily, there aren't any withdrawal symptoms from ADHD medications (for most people), so I was able, with the psychiatrist, to agree on trialling a second medication and start straightaway – no tapering needed. Now this medication has been genuinely like night and day for me, after years and years of struggling, having some stability and then downs that became quite dangerous, feeling something work for me was just amazing. At first, I was wary of how long it would last, I didn't want to get my hopes up after everything I had been through, but I also just knew that this was the one. I made myself think positively and told myself to relax – I had always remained optimistic that I would get there and now I had. I started on a dose of 30mg, and the effects wore off quite quickly (with ADHD meds you should be monitored on a weekly basis until you settle) so I was put up to 50mg and then 60mg and this is where I still am now. This isn't a magic pill – they don't exist

– and it has nothing to do with my ASC, so that way of my brain thinking is still there. Nothing will completely take away the difficulties I have due to being autistic and having ADHD; however, this medication most definitely makes things a lot more manageable for me on a daily basis.

ADHD medications work by helping certain parts of the brain that are underactive/overactive work as they should. For myself, ADHD medication has been the absolute best option and believe me when I say I had tried EVERYTHING else before deciding to go down this route, but having the diagnosis enabled me to understand that there are chemicals in my brain that don't work as well as they should and the medication I now take, helps that. I am (generally) no longer overwhelmed with constant thoughts, I am more motivated, I make more sensible decisions day to day. I have got things done that I had previously put off for years and because of all of this I am happier in general. Having a calmer mind also helps me to keep thinking logically about WHY I am feeling how I am feeling at different times which is super important, so I don't worry unnecessarily. As I've said, there is no such thing as a magic pill and I still have to follow my wellbeing practices and continue to look after myself by sleeping and eating well, but this medication has genuinely helped me to live again and find peace.

The following may trigger others who have struggled with medication withdrawal.

Whilst writing this book, once settled on my ADHD medication for several months, I made the decision, along with the psychiatrist, to come off the anxiety medication that had been prescribed by my GP. This particular medication is notoriously hard to withdraw from and as such you must slowly taper under the guidance of a doctor. I had researched this and was aware of the withdrawal process and side effects. It was my opinion that the anxiety medication had not worked alone, as I had suffered some very low days whilst taking them, and as I have said I'm not a big medication person, so didn't want to be taking something without reason. Now I had my ADHD medication I could get through it and finally move on – little did I know!

At this point I had now been transferred over to the care of the NHS ADHD Team who had also confirmed my diagnosis.

The withdrawal is likened to what heroin addicts feel when they don't have a fix; this is rarely explained to you when you start on these medications; however, if you are at the point where you need to take them, you're more than likely not interested in that anyway – you just desperately want something to help you feel better. My dose was 150mg daily and the plan was to reduce by 37.5mg every two weeks, but within 24 hours I didn't feel right. I didn't feel as 'together' as I had been and my thoughts were all over the place, I also had no appetite whatsoever (not like me). Somehow, I stuck out the taper for six weeks until I was completely without this medication, here are some of the side effects I diarised during this time: constant nausea, flu symptoms, diarrhoea, headaches, feeling weak, shaking, extreme fatigue and constantly wanting to lie down. Along with these, the benefits I had from the ADHD medications for my mind had completely gone, and I was back to where I was at my worst place, I would say even worse as I now had physical symptoms to deal with on top of my mental health. I had lost over a stone, which I don't really have to lose. The ADHD difficulties were back at their worst: overthinking, procrastinating, poor time management, poor sleep patterns, not being able to sit still or read a book as I couldn't focus, and total overwhelm with the whole process. Two days after I took the last pill, the worst started. Without any of the medication in my system at all the withdrawal peaked; genuinely, I have never been so ill in my entire life. I most definitely had a nervous breakdown during this time and the only thing keeping me from going to hospital is the fact that I KNEW that I could have the benefits of the ADHD medication because I had felt it for months. After two weeks without, I had my review with the ADHD team where I told my nurse everything and how every single day for the last two months, more painfully the last two weeks, I had literally just been talking myself through getting through every day. Not surprisingly, my mood was now low, I was emotional, I was not enjoying doing anything that I normally do, even food didn't taste the same, the stimming I do (which I detail in Part Four) had become obsessive at times and I was just so sad because after so many years of feeling overwhelmed, I had finally found something that helped and now it had been taken away. My nurse needed advice from his consultant because I was under the impression that after two weeks completely without, I would be starting to feel better. I didn't want to give up and go back on the medication and to have done all of this for nothing, BUT I didn't know how much longer I could take; I needed an end goal.

It was agreed that I should give it another week; by this point if I still felt as bad, it would not be withdrawal side effects it would be determined that I needed to be back on the anxiety medication. For that week, I was given a 10mg increase in my ADHD medication to see if that would help (it didn't). That week was just as bad as the last with the only difference being that I now had a plan. I'd basically not moved out of my house or wanted to be in anyone's company at all for weeks, I'd just done my best to make it through each day. My first reaction was to be angry that

I had put myself through this in the first place BUT then, and now, I know that I have learned for sure that I need this medication, I am taking it for a reason. It was explained that although the anxiety medication didn't work well alone, it works in conjunction with the ADHD medication which is when I felt the benefits, but when this had been taken away, I was back to square one. So, I started back on the anxiety medication; it took almost two weeks to build back up to the dose I was on originally, but I felt much more like my 'well' self after around a week and it helped that I knew I was on my way to being back to the good place I had been in and moving forward.

I do fully understand some people's aversion to medication and the opinion that people nowadays are just happy to pop a pill and mask their problems. I also agree that some doctors can too easily recommend antidepressants, for example, without fully assessing each patient that they see who says they feel down or overwhelmed. HOWEVER, for some people and for some conditions, medication is not only necessary but vital to help; some will get to a certain point where there is nothing else that will help and there is no other choice.

Strength does not come from winning. Your struggles develop your strengths. When you go through hardships and decide not to surrender, that is strength.

Gandhi

Inspirational Civil Rights Advocate

THE AFTERMATH

The main advantage for me having my diagnoses is that I now know the conditions I have, and I know those conditions inside out, which has helped me manage them and finally understand myself. They are a part of me and always will be and I have accepted that and can always be mindful of that now (as can my family/friends – although I know most don't really 'get it'). It doesn't make me sad or upset at all, I am proud of who I am and having these conditions has been more of a blessing than a curse in many ways. I wasn't ready to work on myself until I was in a comfortable and secure place in my life or until I became a mother. I'm so grateful that I now know how my mind works which is something that not everyone can say. I have absolutely no idea how I have coped, particularly in the last few years. Both my therapist and the psychiatrist who diagnosed me with ADHD, told me it's a miracle that I didn't have a problem with alcohol or drugs to self-medicate, as many people who have lived undiagnosed with ASC and/ or ADHD without support do. I can totally understand this because even for a short time, these substances will make you feel numb and relax your mind; however, in the long run they make things worse. Thankfully, this just wasn't for me, I have never tried a single drug in my life, I've never even been tempted despite often being around people who have done so recreationally. Alcohol has never been my thing either, I will have a couple of drinks maybe twice a year, but I've never really liked the taste or the feeling of being out of control. I can count on just one hand the number of times I've been really drunk in my life.

Ultimately, I think I was forced into realising that I had looked after and worried about everyone else for so long that I needed to look after myself. I think most mums are guilty of that, but sometimes you need to ask yourself – who looks after you? We cannot do it ALL, ALL of the time. I needed to get the right diagnoses instead of it just being passed off as general anxiety when deep down I knew that didn't fit – although my brain was overwhelmed with thoughts, I have never been a worrier as in worrying about accidents or what can go wrong. I needed to learn about and understand myself and to accept who I was, difficulties and all. Having my ADHD diagnosis has enabled me to be prescribed medication that is fitting to my condition. I have worked through my past and present and am ready for my future which I am excited about now that I have clarity and can think straight. I know that, like everyone else, I do and will continue to have bad days, but I also now know that this is normal and nothing that I need to overthink about – asking myself "what's wrong with me?". On these days I need to allow myself time to rest, distract myself, if possible, from my overwhelming thoughts and try my best to think positively. I am of course still learning and will continue to do so, and that is in respect of my own diagnoses and as a parent to a ND child.

Like with mental illness, sometimes being ND can make life feel unmanageable, but I am lucky because I have Jude who brings me happiness every day (not all day every day but every day) and I genuinely don't know where I would be without him. We all need something to believe in and focus on; this really helps. Whether it's family, a career, a passion, religion or spirituality, your future can be positively changed by trusting and believing in something. We all need to enjoy life for what it is, nobody has a totally easy life from start to finish, absolutely everyone struggles at times and experiences loss and sadness, but this is life, so we really need to value the good times and what we have. We also must take care of ourselves, it is our responsibility to do this and only ourselves can do what is needed for each of us to live a happy, healthy life.

Peace is the result of retraining your mind to process life as it is, rather than as you think it should be.

Wayne W. Dyer

Self Help Author and Motivational Speaker

Part Four

The Reality Of Living With ASC And ADHD

HOW ASC AND ADHD AFFECT MY LIFE

Whilst I am genuinely thankful for, and appreciate the way my brain works, there's no denying that day to day life can often be more difficult for those of us who have ASC and/or ADHD than the average person. It's just something we have to learn to live with and do our best with. The fact that, currently, most people don't understand (or even believe in) our conditions make things harder. I hope this will change for the better in the future and that the wider society appreciates that not all disabilities, conditions or illnesses are visible, and just because you may not understand them personally doesn't mean they don't exisist.

You can't tell by looking at me or Jude that we are ND; I feel this is a blessing and a curse. A blessing because in most cases we don't want to be treated differently (or to be felt sorry for) BUT it's a curse because nobody has a clue how hard we work every single day or how our conditions affect us – this means that any necessary provisions and/or allowances are not given unless we explicitly ask for them or explain – which usually wouldn't always be the case if you could SEE our diagnoses. Like many people with ASC and/or ADHD I also live with autoimmune diseases, mine being Fibromyalgia and Crohn's Disease. Again, these illnesses are lifelong and will never be cured, and they are invisible. I know that most people who suffer with these conditions struggle with the fact that outwardly they look healthy and 'normal', but they are often exhausted and always aware in their mind that they have an incurable illness which isn't easy. Again, it's not about wanting sympathy but wanting some understanding from those around them – which you are more likely to get if you have a visible illness. I absolutely hate to moan about anything I struggle with, especially to my husband who I see every day, it makes you feel like you're always complaining and you're overly aware that this can be draining for the other person too.

It is extremely hard to describe exactly how it feels to be ND, in my case to have ASC and ADHD, but I will try my best to do it justice in the hope that other ND people reading this can see that they're not alone and that there are other people who relate – although we're all different a lot of what we experience is similar. Also, I hope that it helps NT readers in some way to understand what we live with.

This is just how it is for me.

"The swan glides on the surface of the pond, looking calm and in control. Yet underneath the water it's a different story, feet frantically paddling away."

Personally, I would say that having ADHD affects my day-to-day life more than being autistic. ASC is more prevalent in social situations and issues with change, which as an adult I can manage quite well given the fact that I can control, mostly, where I am, who I'm with and what I'm doing. Whereas I can't escape my mind, and this is what ADHD controls. My mind NEVER has a break and when I say that I don't mean most days or when I have a particularly busy day, or when I'm stressed, I mean from the minute I wake up to the minute I (make myself) fall asleep I am thinking, constantly, every day, and it's been that way for as long as I can remember. This has been the most difficult part for me during my struggles in recent years as it becomes completely overwhelming and unbearable at times. These thoughts can be ideas, of which I have many – a lot that never get acted upon because it would be physically impossible. It is often thoughts about what I need/want to do, today, tomorrow, next week, next year, in 20 years, the list goes on. Thoughts completely unrelated to whatever it is that I am doing at that moment in time, the same goes for memories. A conversation I had 20 years ago, something I watched on the television four years ago, a meal I ate six months ago, or something I read 30 years ago, all can and do pop into my head at any minute of the day amidst everything else, again nothing at all relevant to what I'm already thinking or doing at the time.

Again, I do know that it's hard for anyone who doesn't experience this to completely understand, but believe me when I say it is EXHAUSTING. This is one of the main reasons I find that I can sometimes become irritable, it's like I'm concentrating on a thousand things 24/7 so when someone talks to me or calls me and I'm not expecting it or ready for it, it rudely interrupts me as if someone is interrupting a conversation – although logically I do know the other person isn't aware of that. I'm not being cold, I know it comes across like that most of the time because usually I can't hide it well, I just physically can't help it. I used to worry more about what people thought of me but now I completely accept myself for who I am (and have made the people in my life aware of my diagnoses) and if they don't understand me, or even try to, then quite frankly that's their problem.

Along with the constant thinking, I am always, also visually overwhelmed – things NT people don't see or really notice, I will. For example, if there is an odd number of items on the shelf at the supermarket, if there is a missing placemat on the table in a restaurant, patterns in wallpaper, words in car registration plates or a crack in a tile. My eyes take everything in all the time no matter where I am or whatever else I am doing. However, like most ND traits, this can also be a skill, having a good eye for detail.

It's not just my visual senses that are heightened; for example, if I visit someone whose television is too loud it physically hurts my ears. I'm also super sensitive to smells, I cannot stomach car air fresheners, I can smell someone's perfume a mile away and it will make me nauseous if it's too strong, and I can literally smell things I've cooked at home for days after.

It is constant overwhelming overwhelm; it may be helpful if you can imagine – sitting in a room with 20 televisions on the highest volume, ten radios playing different songs, being on a phone call trying to take directions whilst driving, having ten different web pages open on your laptop and trying to place urgent orders on them all at once, five people asking you important questions (most of which you don't understand completely and need more detail on), feeling so cold it's uncomfortable and being unable to get warm, feeling happy, stressed, excited and frustrated all at the same time, being so tired you could drop but physically not being able to sit still and rest, having the feeling that you have forgotten something but not knowing what it is, replaying an argument you had with someone months ago, thinking about what to get your partner for their birthday, thinking if your child is doing ok at school, suddenly replaying a pointless conversation from 15 years ago in your head, wondering if you are getting enough sleep and eating healthily enough, having painfully restless legs, your clothes being uncomfortable, impulsively counting the tiles on the floor and creating a series of patterns in your head, feeling impatient because you can't do EVERYTHING at once. All whilst completing an exam that has to be finished in five minutes and stressing that you have to leave the house for an important doctor's appointment in two minutes and it's never going to happen – AGAIN.

Again, this is not an exaggeration, this is what our ADHD world is like all day every day. Of course, what we think about and experience changes from person to person and as we grow, and our life evolves, but the consistency is always there and for some it's much worse than others. And remember we have to learn from childhood to live like this because of course as a child and young adult you don't know that this isn't how everyone else lives or how to express it. Alongside this overwhelm that we face constantly, we also have to pretend to be like 'everyone else', to hide what we like, what we don't like, what we're feeling, thinking, hearing and seeing so that we 'fit in'.

I hope this will help some people understand better why we need some space, why we sometimes need quiet time alone, why we need to be given a break and/or allowances to be made in certain situations and why it's fine for us to need to move around or 'stim' to self-regulate. Also, this is one of the reasons why we often tend to like a plan. I need a plan and to prepare for everything I do – I wish I didn't because it's just more work – but if I don't, I feel painfully uncomfortable. I hope in the future that ND children don't have to hide or 'mask' who they are and can live as openly and as freely as they wish, without judgement or exclusion.

Of course as adults, on top of all the above, we also have to manage our everyday lives like everyone else, including but not exclusive to our children, our partners, our jobs, our families, friends, our health, thinking about our appearance in an ever-increasingly superficial world, looking after our home – the list goes on. This is often a lot for most NT people so try and imagine managing this alongside experiencing life the way that we do. This is one reason that some ND people choose not to have families or partners or just don't get to that point – much like I explained how I feel like I have chosen not to have many friends – because it can simply be too much. Of course, there are NT people who also choose not to 'settle down' or have children because they don't want to be committed or responsible for anyone else. I understand both, and as I detailed earlier for a long time never thought I would have a family; however, I am so glad I did!

When most people (particularly women) are stressed out, frustrated, upset, angry or on the edge, they will usually reach out to their friends/family/colleagues to 'moan' and let off steam as everyone around them goes through similar times, BUT when you're ND this is something else we miss out on because we have nobody to discuss our issues with – in most cases not a single person we know, or who we know well, has any idea what it's like to live with our brains working the way they do. Simply NOBODY 'gets it'.

It is genuinely like being from another planet and kind of learning as we go what is 'normal' and having lives with these other species but always being on the outside, never being understood or truly known inside and out. If you're ND and you have a person/people in your life that genuinely want to know EVERYTHING about how it feels – how your mind works, what you see, what you hear, how you interpret things differently to them – and they ask truly interested questions and try their best to educate themselves to be able to support you and live alongside you in the best way they can, then you are extremely lucky and have someone special.

Although this is how it should be – because everyone deserves to be treated with love and understanding and to be accepted for who they are – it is often not the case, but I do hope that as generations evolve it will be more common and the positive effects of that will be amazing.

Of course, even with medication some days are more difficult than others; for example, if I have PMT or haven't slept well. I sometimes find school holidays quite hard because of the element of change to my daily routine and if I have a lot to do, I obviously don't have as much time to get things done – which creates a vicious circle as I'll then stay up later than I should to get everything finished but then I don't get enough sleep which worsens the overthinking and procrastinating and I end up overwhelmed with a backlog of jobs to do. I am working on planning things better in advance of such times. As I have mentioned, medication has greatly improved many things for me and has brought a lot more 'peace' to my mind and allowed me to think logically about how I can make things easier for myself and I will continue to work on this to improve my quality of life.

I also want to point out that this is how I feel as a grown woman and a mother to a non-verbal ND child; it was not **as** difficult (for me) when I was a child or in my younger years – although I have felt different in every room I've been in in my entire life.

As I have mentioned, as life gets more stressful, being undiagnosed manifests into something we cannot sustain forever and something must give, usually our health, and we HAVE to ask for help, get support and look after ourselves better. Anyone can feel sorry for themselves, but I don't see the point in that...that isn't going to help anyone, least not ourselves. Like anyone with struggles, it is OUR choice to pick ourselves up and create the life that we want.

Resolve to be thyself and know that he who finds himself loses his misery

Matthew Arnold

Historical Poet

LIVING WITH ASC/ADHD

Further to the above, I want to share details of what I find most difficult in the hope that it can help others who relate.

- Being misunderstood is probably one of the biggest ways in which my conditions negatively affect my life. Any NT person can simply not understand how it feels to live with a ND mind. I would love to be able to let the people around me live with my mind for one day and see how they feel afterwards – obviously this isn't possible, which is a shame. For people to understand and learn they need to want to, and sadly most people don't, or at least not until they have a more personal connection like having a child who is ND, for example.

- The routines I have to follow more often than not make me late, for example if we oversleep for school,

I couldn't just throw on some clothes and rush out of the door. I could never leave the house without making the beds, there can be no dishes out in the kitchen or any mess at all, everything has to be in its place, or I physically couldn't leave. This and poor time awareness are the main reasons why it is extremely hard for me to have to be anywhere for a specific time.

- If I have appointments or plans, I usually get anxious about them and would rather not go even if I know I will enjoy myself and be happy I went. If I have one appointment or plan that will take over the whole day for me and I will think about it for days in advance.

- My inability to be spontaneous and deviate from my plans or routine is very difficult, which is hard when others are involved as it can come across as selfish to NT people. I also am not a fan of surprises and would always rather choose my own gift or plan my own event. I know this is something that most people think is thoughtful, so I do get this can be hard for others to understand.

- Because of constantly overthinking, I have terrible trouble relaxing, I find it almost impossible to sit still and just 'be'. I ALWAYS have to be doing something. Even if I'm driving, I don't want to just sit in quiet or waste time, I will have to make any phone calls I need to make or clean inside my car. I physically cannot lie/sit down and do nothing. With ADHD it often feels almost as if we're more 'at rest' if we're doing something. On the rare occasions I do sit doing nothing, it feels uneasy to me like I've forgotten something, my brain panics and will automatically start running through a list of things that I should be doing or what I should be thinking about.

- Because my brain is constantly working overtime and I don't sit still, I often feel exhausted later in the day because I quite literally burn out.

- Particularly in recent years given (the increasingly negative) ongoing world affairs, I must limit what I read or watch as the strong sense of injustice that I have, and my sense of empathy can completely consume me. Having such empathy is a blessing and a curse. Many people think that those who have ADHD and/or ASC lack empathy (this is particularly thought of about autistic people); however, this is a myth. Those of us with these conditions can often feel empathy much more acutely than NT people. I want to help everyone in need, particularly children. I literally become obsessed with thinking of ways in which I can save people in every situation I hear about, which of course isn't possible unfortunately.

- I hate to be cold and will shut down if I get really uncomfortable with the temperature. By shutdown I mean it becomes very difficult for me to communicate. If I am stuck somewhere in (what feels to me like) the extremes. I feel the cold terribly and always have to have my house warm, if I'm somewhere I can't control the temperature I will have to comment on it or keep my coat on and I automatically sit tensed up, hating every second.

- I HATE flying, this is a problem that is getting worse with age and something I am trying to control. I will literally shut down from everything and everyone around me before boarding a plane and for most of the flight. I have tried medication in the past, but nothing really helps. I'm not afraid of crashing, it's more the fact that I can't stop the plane and get off if I wanted to. It's claustrophobic, you're trapped thousands of miles high in the air with no control whatsoever. Then the noises that I don't understand and possible turbulence, it's A LOT and I just do what I can to get through it every time. If I didn't love holidays so much, I wouldn't bother.

- My need for 'sameness' is probably boring to most other people, but I just like what I know and don't need to change or try new things frequently. Since I was a child even the end of a weekend or a holiday has always brought me an uneasy feeling because there is going to be a change to the routine again.

- I will eat/drink mostly anything and everything; however, it is the way in which things are prepared that I have trouble with. For example, my husband who I have been with for more than 13 years has probably made me five cups of tea in all that time because I just HAVE to do it myself. If someone offered to make me a sandwich, I would have to tell them exactly how to do it so I may as well just do it myself and that's the case for most things in my life.

- I am hypermobile which is common in ASC. This means that my joints bend further than they should which with age causes some painful conditions such as Fibromyalgia, which causes me to have aching joints most days.

- I often can't control myself in a conversation with others and can speak over people, it's like I'm watching myself in slow motion, but I just cannot help it.

- I also never really know if I'm saying the right thing in conversation or if I'm being totally inappropriate, especially if I don't think before I speak.

- I am also aware that I 'dump' information onto people and when the person on the receiving end isn't interested in whatever I'm offloading about, but again I can't help it. I also often 'interview' people that I am in conversation with as in I will bombard them with questions as if I'm going to forget what I want to ask (which can and does happen).

- Over the course of my life, I have subconsciously learned to make myself give people eye contact when I'm speaking with them, although it isn't comfortable for me, I know it's what's deemed as 'appropriate'. However, the more comfortable I am with the person I find I don't make myself do this as much.

- I often get lost in my own thoughts and can find it hard to pay attention to things or other people.

- I feel most at ease when I don't have to make myself communicate like a NT person. I love being at home in my bubble where I can completely be myself.

- I often feel like people are watching me to see if I am behaving 'correctly' even though they're probably not; like I've said, I have always been overly aware of other people's opinions which in general I don't care about, but I don't like the thought of being watched as it makes me self-conscious.

- I do not handle criticism at all well and can become very defensive even if it is just someone else's idea of a joke. I am VERY easy to 'wind up' and have been the same since I was a child. Autistic people often take things literally and/or don't 'get' NT humour, which doesn't help.

- I don't like unplanned visits at home, I do like hosting for the children in our house but struggle with things being moved out of place and the mess this can cause. If I'm prepared, I know and can plan for that, but short notice I'm not great with. Again, I know this can make me look rude to others.

- If have taken too much on or am more stressed than normal, I need quite a lot of quiet time and alone time to organise my thoughts as they become overwhelming. Also, if I am visiting someone else or on the rare occasion I am socialising, I will sometimes have to take myself off to another room just to be alone for a while because I get overwhelmed. I also catch myself pacing in a room whilst I am running through the checklists in my head as it seems to help rather than just being stood or sat still; this is a self-regulating behaviour.

- I have to sleep in complete darkness and with earplugs as I can't stand any light or noise at all when I am trying to sleep. A NT person may think a room is dark and quiet – to most ND people it won't be! I have a full sleep kit beside my bed.

- I'm not great at sensory multi-tasking, for example, if I am on the phone ordering a takeaway and my husband shouts what he wants I physically can't listen to the two different voices and get very frustrated.

- I can be impatient (I HATE to wait in traffic, for example) probably because I'm no good at sitting still. Even having my nails done is difficult. I know most people find this relaxing or a treat, but to me it's just a necessity and not something I enjoy.

- If something isn't written down I will forget it, probably because my mind is so full, but my long-term memory is great.

- I get little obsessions which can lead me to going down a Google rabbit hole until all hours of the night. For example, if I watch a new TV show or read a new book that I'm really into, I'll want to know everything about the characters, actors, authors etc immediately. This usually lasts a few days.

- I'm not good with last minute plans, whatever it is, it takes a lot of effort, planning and preparation for myself and/or Jude to go out, so I make plans well in advance. If people change plans last minute, I honestly can't explain the frustration I feel and the effort I then have to make, to rearrange, change my diary, change the to-do lists on my phone, explaining the changes to Jude etc.

- Waking up has ALWAYS been an issue for me. I don't know if it's a sensory thing or because I just loved my bed!

- Particularly if I'm stressed or under pressure, I will calm myself by 'stimming', using my phone quite impulsively. I follow a sequence to check my emails, social media, bank app, texts, photos, WhatsApp messages, calls and internet. It is physically uncontrollable and something I have to do to stay calm.

- I'm quite good with directions but cannot grasp any part of geography. I genuinely have no idea where most places are in the world.

- I physically cannot stand loud people, or cars or anything loud really, although, in certain settings such as a bar, I may enjoy loud music – but of course this will be planned in advance, and I will be prepared for it. You will often find that autistic children themselves may be loud, but don't like being around other loud people. This is because the way in which we process senses is different to NT people.

- I often have no concept of time, especially when I'm 'hyper' focused on something – my husband often has to come and tell me what time it is. This also doesn't help my problem with lateness.

Happiness can only exist in acceptance

George Orwell

Historical Poet

STRATEGIES I HAVE LEARNED TO HELP MANAGE MY DIFFICULTIES

The good news is, living with ASC/ADHD can be managed to make things easier for us – but we have to be proactive in this. Some of these are things I've done my whole adult life before I even knew I was autistic or had ADHD. They are ways in which I naturally learned to cope with how my brain works. Some are things I've started to do in the last couple of years, since my diagnoses, which have really helped me to manage my life better and to be generally happier and healthier. A few years before my diagnoses, I was told by a therapist that I should try to get out of the habit I had of keeping daily to-do lists and writing things down so much. However, the psychiatrist who diagnosed my ADHD actually told me that this is one of the strategies they recommend, to help newly diagnosed people.

I hope that some of you reading may find them useful too.

- For peace of mind, I keep a daily to-do list on my phone for each day of the week. I include simple things such as getting dressed and times that I need to follow, like what time we have to leave for school – this is helpful just to have as a backup – I obviously know I have to get dressed every day and what time my son needs to be in school for, but when you have a mind that is constantly overwhelmed, it's always good to have something to look at to guide you. This eases the pressure and reduces overwhelm. I also have all my notes backed up in case I lose my phone – this has happened on occasion and has been traumatic.

- I cannot stress the importance of planning, preparing, and organising for people who are ND. It helps limit the overwhelm you feel and prevents last minute rushing around which sends us spiralling. Just make sure you set REALISTIC timeframes for your plans.

- I have alarms set on my phone every day to remind me of when I need to leave for school, taking my meds, appointments and even eating and giving myself time to get ready etc. This helps me be prepared so I don't get as stressed or anxious about the time because nobody is more aware of my lateness than me.

- Each day I go through my to-do list for the next day and include details such as what I may need to take with me to any appointments or meetings. How long I will need to get ready, how long it will take to get there etc. I then set my alarms ready for the next day. It helps me to be prepared by knowing what's happening the next day.

- Once a week I sit and go through my diary for the following week to add any appointments etc to my daily to-do lists. I can then prepare anything needed and have in my mind a plan of what is next.

- I keep an original list on my phone for the general things I have to do every day to cut and paste for the next week and then I add anything extra around those things. This just means I don't have to try and remember it all and type it out again.

- I also use the notes app on my phone to write down any thoughts I have that I don't want to forget. As ND people literally have non-stop thoughts and ideas, we can also forget them in a second and some of these thoughts and ideas are important and amazing!

- I will extensively prepare notes for any meetings I have, such as a meeting with Jude's school, so I don't forget what I want to discuss. It's easy to get overwhelmed when talking to professionals but, especially with regards to your child, you know them best and what they're capable of, so you need to prepare.

- I have lists for everything in my diary such as my housework routine, laundry days, what things I need to check to put on my food shopping list and even what I need to do to prepare for going on holiday and preparing for Christmas. Again, this is helpful for me as my brain is already so full that having things written down means I won't forget anything and therefore won't stress about that – it gives me peace of mind.

- I couldn't even begin to go into any shop without a list, it boggles my mind how people can do this! I do a food shopping list every week and plan our meals for every day the following week and all the ingredients needed for them, so I know well in advance what is needed, what I'm cooking and what we'll be eating. All preparation is super helpful.

- I make sure I spread my jobs out for the week so I don't get overwhelmed on each day, so I will do my laundry and housework one day, diary planning another day, food shopping another. I will then plan any appointments, meetings, or work around these, always careful to not book too much in to one day. I learned this by burning myself out trying to do too much on a daily basis. This would then end in me moving jobs to the next day and so on and it would just snowball and then I would be awake until all hours finishing things –which doesn't help my mind at all.

- Recently, I have found that it can be beneficial to me to – for at least part of the day when I don't have any specific plans – not to use my phone notes and to wake up and potter about at home without being restricted to a schedule. I definitely couldn't do this every day, or if I was to leave my house, but it's been nice to try something different.

- Following on from this I can't emphasise enough how important sleep is for those who are ND. Unfortunately, people with ASC/ADHD often struggle with sleep but we must try to figure out what is the best way for ourselves to get a good rest as not doing so makes our symptoms so much more unbearable. There is more advice on this in the Helpful Tips section.

- I am trying to do better at not taking too much on as this most certainly does not help with being overwhelmed and my poor concept of time means I think I can fit more into a day than I can!

- If someone tells me something I need to remember, I will ask them to text me if I can't write it down in that moment as I will forget. If I do forget something I know I have and then it plays on my mind constantly.

- I have self-care basics that I must do every day as part of my routine, these really make a positive difference to my wellbeing and if it's not planned it doesn't happen, so remember when planning your day to include time for yourself! More details in the Helpful Tips section.

- At least once a week I make sure I have a quiet hour to myself to practise positive thinking. One, to know that I have this time so don't need to overthink on other days, and two, to make sure I'm on track for all my goals etc – such as reviewing how I'm feeling with regards to my meds, do I need a catch up with my GP or ADHD nurse? Do I feel happy, if not, why not, and what can I do about it? Is Jude happy, are we doing everything we can for him? Finances, relationship, future plans etc. In CBT this is described as scheduling 'time to worry' which I know sounds crazy but it really helps if you know you have that time to think things through so you can try and push it to the back of your mind if you're overthinking these issues constantly. Sometimes if I am feeling stressed, I will have a little time each day to quickly think over these areas so I can remind myself I don't need to worry.

- Something else I've learned to do is to block negative or intrusive thoughts. Naturally we all have these thoughts but they're not useful and can give someone who is ND even more to think about unnecessarily, so it's best to not dwell on them and totally block them if they pop into your head, or to switch to a positive thought or memory. You would be surprised how easily you can pick this up once you focus on doing it – and you can train your brain at any age.

- Once a month I get quite a strong massage to help with my joint pain and it's also an hour where I have no choice but to lie still and rest. I would recommend this to anyone who has frequent aches/pains. I also use a brace to help with the tension in my shoulders.

- I try to have an afternoon most weeks, when one of our mums picks up Jude from school, to purposefully not make any plans and practise some self-care, have an early bath and TRY to relax. I also luckily get a lie in every Sunday as Shaun takes Jude out to see his grandma. I make sure I catch up on my sleep, which is something I look forward to every single week. When you're ND and/or have autoimmune conditions, you really need to look after yourself and sleep is the best prevention and cure for everything!

- Therapy is, in my opinion, one of the best things you can do if you feel you need some support or you have issues you need help with. Personally, and as a couple, if you have a good therapist it can be life changing.

- I do love my chocolate and cake, but generally I try to eat well. This is both good for my energy levels and Crohn's Disease.

- Music is, and always has been a big part of my life. I can't sing a note or play an instrument, but I have always listened to music to help me feel good. To dance to, get excited to, feel energised with, to feel understood or even to cry to. Without even knowing it, you can take a break from your thoughts when you're listening to music. Research shows how important music is to our wellbeing.

- Being self-aware and looking after yourself is highly important. Nobody knows how you feel, physically or mentally, other than you. And unfortunately, we don't have medical professionals who can check in with us and see how we're doing regularly – we need to do it ourselves, especially if we have medical conditions.

- I have learned to use the brain I have been given to my advantage. I hyperfocus to learn about the things I am passionate about and interested in. Having something that you're genuinely interested in, to do on a daily basis, helps you be thankful for the way your mind works. Having gratitude for our differences is very helpful for our journey.

- I make goals for myself and write them down in lots of detail, which gives me something to work towards – even subconsciously – and achieving goals is such a positive thing. I also make realistic deadlines for these goals (even if they are years in advance) because otherwise there isn't really anything to properly aim for. Visualising or manifesting is not about hoping to win the lottery, for example; it changes your outlook and behaviours that enable you to create opportunities for yourself. I really believe we can write our own life story; we don't have to just accept what we're given or what society tells us we should or shouldn't be doing.

- Keeping a positive mindset is essential to everyone, but to those of us with conditions that often come with mental health issues, we have to take control of our own thoughts as much as possible, so we don't spiral. As I have mentioned, it is possible to teach yourself quite quickly to replace negative thoughts with positive ones.

- I'm trying to do better at listening to my body. If you need to rest, rest even for ten minutes to catch your breath. Your body will tell you what you need and if you don't listen it will force you to eventually.

- I have learned to focus on my breath if I feel myself getting worked up or anxious as this helps calm us down and brings us back to the present. I find that taking several breaths in, counting to three and then breathing out counting to four really helps.

- I am continually working on reminding myself not to feel guilty about needing time, understanding, space, or for looking after myself. I am a mother but if I don't look after myself, I will be of no use to my son now or in the future. I am also modelling to him the positive ways in which he can practise self-care and manage any difficulties his conditions may bring.

My Daily Routine Basics

- As soon as I wake up, I play some positive affirmations and do some quick yoga stretches.

- I get everything ready for Jude, help him get ready and off to school.

- I will take my meds usually early morning but, if I have plans that I need to be motivated for later in the day I will take them slightly later.

- I will make myself have some breakfast before my meds. Some ADHD medication affects your appetite and mine does so I have to eat before I'm no longer hungry. I'm not a big fan of breakfast but I usually have two boiled eggs as that's good for my protein intake. I will usually have something light for lunch.

- I'll take some vitamins and the rest throughout the day as some aren't ideal to mix (such as Vitamin C with my ADHD meds). Magnesium I take before bed as it helps with sleep.

- I make sure to do my Pilates and guided meditation early on whilst I have more energy, because if I put it off until later, experience has taught me, I won't do it and I feel so much better for the rest of the day if I have done this.

- Every day I have out a two-litre bottle of water (with cordial as I just can't drink water alone) which makes me drink it throughout the day. Otherwise, I just never get thirsty.

- I get done any work/chores etc I have to do as early in the day as possible, again because later in the day I won't have the motivation.

- I spend time with Jude after school and we have some family time relaxing before dinner.

- After dinner I will write my gratitude and positivity journals.

- After bath time and before bedtime I will play some positive affirmations and do some yoga stretches.

- I will generally try to practise some visualisation while I go to sleep and find playing beach wave sounds helps me relax.

Take pride in how far you've come. Have faith in how far you can go.

Michael Josephson

Professor and Charity Founder

NEURODIVERGENT WOMEN

Depending on who is reading this, this is either a popular or unpopular opinion...in general, life is harder for women. Whilst positive change is being made and things are moving in the right direction, women have struggled with inequality and discrimination for centuries. We live in a man's world and whether consciously or not we are deemed as secondary in every aspect of it. The pressures on us both in our smaller societies and the bigger world are huge, especially in our modern world with all the ideals of perfection.

As previously mentioned, partly due to the differences within our brains, far fewer females are diagnosed with ASC/ADHD than males, although we now know that this isn't the case. Most are not diagnosed until later in life after their child is diagnosed or as a result of extreme struggles with hormonal fluctuations and/or menopause.

We go unnoticed for much longer partly because we have the ability to mask our traits to the outside world, and our symptoms often present differently and more subtly than ND males. There is therefore currently less information about ND women as we have been much less studied, but that is changing.

For many females in the developed world, we are steered towards taking a contraceptive pill from an age when our bodies and hormones are still developing, the result of which (physical issues aside) often cause structural changes within our brain. Our brains, and bodies, eventually have to acclimatise to not having these hormones once we either stop taking the pill due to deciding to have a child or as we age – which is recommended by our doctors. Naturally we produce less testosterone than males – testosterone is a hormone which, amongst other things, helps dictate your mood, motivation and libido. Generally speaking, females live with hormone difficulties from our teenage years through to our fifties. We go through puberty, beginning menstruation, hormonal fluctuations due to this, pregnancy, and age. Recently it has been learned that ADHD is hugely affected by our hormones – particularly with regards to PMT and menopause. These times can literally make ND women feel suicidal one day and fine the next for no other reason than the hormonal changes within our bodies.

This information needs to be highlighted to ND women and more research done, as well as more training given to GPs, to help the women who struggle significantly with these issues to find a treatment most beneficial to them to enable them to live a healthier and happier life. In my opinion, all girls should be educated about their hormones, how best to keep them healthy and the common issues we face as we grow. As a result, this will also positively reflect on our children, families and relationships, as well as being what we deserve. Like many other things, do we think that after centuries of struggles with menopause there still wouldn't be any better, easier, more accessible treatments if it was men that went through this?

The good news is that there are treatments that can help us, but like most things surrounding ASC/ADHD we have to find it and ask for it ourselves. Alongside dietary and lifestyle changes, there are hormone supplements and medications that can make things at least more bearable. After what I have learned recently during the very beginning of my own perimenopause journey, I would highly recommend requesting at least annual blood tests to check your hormone and thyroid levels once you reach your forties – again, this is something you will have to be proactive about to look after yourself as this isn't something that is offered routinely.

For any women that feel they could possibly have ASC there is a very detailed resource available – search online for 'Samantha Craft's Unofficial Checklist' - which lists many of the traits that affect females, in particular.

On a personal note, I would really like any woman struggling with these and other issues to know that although you feel alone, you are not. There are thousands of women just like you, I am one of them, and there is help available and many things that you can do to help yourself. And, rightly or wrongly, we do have to help ourselves. We have to use our strength to look after ourselves and find the right way for us. We also need to ignore the negative narrative that some people have with regards to the new generation of women who are speaking out on this subject as if it is wrong to do so. Everyone is entitled to their own opinion, and I agree that we don't need to shout and scream about our private lives; however, we also shouldn't feel like it's a taboo subject when literally every woman on the planet goes through it to varying degrees.

There are many confidential forums online where you can discuss your issues with other women and gain support and advice – I have provided some sites on the Recommended Resources section.

There is no limit to what we, as women, can acclomplish

Michelle Obama

Author and Former First Lady of the USA

MY JOURNEY

Although I have finally found medication that helps me, and feel better than I have in years, I am not 'cured'. I will always be autistic, and I will always have ADHD and because of that my brain will always work differently to most other people – I will live with that for the rest of my life, which I have accepted. In times of stress or hormonal changes, or sometimes for no apparent reason at all, I know that I will still have bad days. Anyone who is ND or suffers with their mental health will have to accept this, BUT we can learn what to do during these times to help it pass easier, and I can't stress enough the importance of having a healthy lifestyle and keeping a positive mindset. Building a life that makes you genuinely happy, makes it ALL worth it and you have to be 100% honest with yourself and self-aware to live the best life you can for you. For example, it has been helpful for me to learn why I feel so overwhelmed when my normal routine is disrupted. I love Christmas time BUT the lack of routine and changes to daily life mean it does reach a point where I feel things get a bit much. In the past I hadn't understood this or made the connection and put more pressure on myself for not feeling as happy as I 'should' be during this festive time. However, now I can prepare myself and think logically about why I feel overwhelmed and tell myself it will pass.

I know lots of people wonder what the benefit is of being diagnosed later in life, why would you bother? You've managed until this stage in life, what's the point? First of all, I couldn't manage any longer. After everything I learned about ASC through my son, I just knew it was a part of me and I wanted the official diagnosis. After several years, of being told I was 'just' suffering with general anxiety, I finally got confirmation that the fact I KNEW I wasn't, was correct. The issue was/is that my mind does not stop, it is constantly working overtime, I find it hard to relax and just be or enjoy what is happening around me because my thoughts are constant and it's impossible to just switch them off. The funny thing is that when you are diagnosed later in life your autistic/ADHD traits often become more obvious than they were before – the main reason for this is that you now know who you are and why you are how you are, and you stop trying to mask and 'fit in', you can breathe and just be yourself, which is liberating.

I also now know why I have always felt different and am assured that there isn't anything 'wrong with me', my brain just works differently to those who are NT, it always has, and it always will. I don't think having my diagnoses has changed me other than it has made me more assured and feel the freedom to be myself. Shaun says that, to him, I had always been a bit 'different', but he's always liked that. Every single one of us has some issues/quirks, many struggle with addiction, mental health, poor physical health and weight problems – this is the reality of life.

I also wanted to be able to tell Jude that I understand him and that we're both ND and that it is absolutely fine to be different and in fact a gift. It breaks my heart to see the number of ND children and young people who struggle so much with not having the answers to why they feel so different that they feel like they don't want to live. Hopefully as awareness grows around ASC and ADHD, the time it takes to be diagnosed will drastically improve and the negative stigma will be a thing of the past.

Personally, I would always recommend looking into getting a diagnosis even if it's just for you to know for yourself. Particularly for women as we get older, and our hormones change (detailed more in the section 'Neurodivergent Women'). Many people who are late diagnosed go through a period of grief and anger. Angry that they weren't supported and diagnosed earlier and how that could have been better for their lives, and grieving for the person they had thought they were. I do understand this but for me it would have been impossible to have an earlier diagnosis as there just was not the awareness when I was younger and I'm actually happier now that I know who I am.

I'm genuinely glad that my brain works how it does or I would never have achieved all that I have. My ability to 'hyper focus' has enabled me to ensure that my son has the best support possible and for him to be tremendously happy despite his communication difficulties; as I said, we ALL have our own strengths and weaknesses, and this is mine. I know that I have changed as a result of all that I have discovered about myself but only for the better. I would never have achieved the personal growth and understanding of myself had I not made the choice to take control of my life. Over the last few years, I think we can all agree that the world has changed and we, as a society, have changed with it, whether we have wanted to or not. Only we ourselves can make the change positive or let it consume us.

For those of us who are deep thinkers, or have a strong sense of injustice, it can seem like everyone else seems ok with the (seemingly increasing) negativity of our world and we can't understand that. People all too often seem like they're out to get each other or outdo each other and we don't want to be a part of that, and the only way I've learned to deal with that is to try not to see it. I genuinely don't understand how everyone doesn't get as outraged as I do when there are such awful things happening every day. Unfortunately, we can't change the world and we can't change other people, but what we CAN do is make our own little worlds as positive and fulfilling as possible and to help others when we can. Of course, we need to keep having truthful conversations and supporting and advocating for what we believe in, but we can't let it affect us negatively when things are way out of our control.

I recently read these words written by Steven Bartlett – who is an influential young entrepreneur whose work I have been a fan of for a long time (details in the Recommended Resources section) – and I think they're fitting:

> "Everyone seems to be getting prettier on the outside but uglier on the inside"

I am not perfect, and of course I have made mistakes in life, but that is how we learn. In hindsight, and with the knowledge I now have, I have at times acted impulsively and not thought things through in certain situations or with certain choices I have made; however, I have never intentionally hurt anyone and continue to work on doing better, giving back, and working on being the best version of myself possible. I also have absolutely no regrets and have always lived by this because it's just common sense to me that there is absolutely no point in wishing things had been different because there is no way to change the past, it's impossible.

Writing this book has been extremely difficult for me at times. Naturally I always put a lot of pressure on myself, but with this I really wanted to get it right because the subject is so important to me. During some parts of the process, I have had issues with my medication, which as I have detailed were a big struggle, but I wanted to continue writing through it so I could be as honest as possible about how it felt and what I was going through, in the hope that it might help someone else. I've had to revisit my childhood which I didn't enjoy and then having to write continuously about the difficulties you have or have had and any negative experiences, makes you focus on them more which in an ideal world I wouldn't have had to do – however, I will now work to move on and heal from putting myself under a microscope.

Throughout this whole journey of my mental health, diagnoses, acceptance, and medication, what has kept me going is the fact that I wanted to take control of my life and understand completely, who I was and why. Following on from that I could then figure out where I wanted to go and what happiness was FOR ME and what I needed to do to finally feel at peace. The longer time has gone on the more I wanted to keep going to have a better understanding for my son and to raise awareness for others with ASC/ADHD in their lives. I have learned to look after myself and make choices to keep my distance from some people because you can't change a person or the past, but you can choose to move on. There are people whom it is not possible to completely lose contact with, so I just limit the amount of time I spend around them, if I don't feel good being in their company, or afterwards, then I won't force myself to make the effort; some people are just not compatible and that's fine.

Now at almost 40 years young I finally know who I am and the life I want; age means nothing to me, so I know I still have my whole life ahead of me which I'm excited about. I want to continue being self-aware and achieving everything that I have planned. I want to continue to help Jude live the best life possible – which is limitless. Writing this has been therapeutic for my past and I am happy to have fulfilled a lifelong goal of mine, as a child I loved to read and write and dreamed of writing books. I am grateful every day for my life and how far I have come.

Personally, a big goal of mine is to help people in my local community on a much bigger platform than what is currently possible. I would love to help other people with ASC and/or ADHD across all ages and gender, and their families. I believe with every part of me that anything is possible if you put your mind to it, so I'm going to continue working towards that. Also, I really want to help children in need – there is nothing more important than our children. I recently adopted my husband's nan as my own – she has dementia and as her condition deteriorated it became impossible for her to live alone and care for herself. I helped her daily for several months whilst a suitable care home was found and although it did have a stressful impact on my life, being involved in this was a real education for me. We have gained a very close bond and I visit her weekly and always make sure her needs are being met – something I have promised her I will always do. Our relationship has also helped me, I have always been drawn to older people and think they're the most interesting of people with amazing experience. Making a difference to someone's life in such an intimate way, has assured me that I definitely want to be a part of helping others in the future.

As part of my ongoing wellbeing journey, I have a goal to visit one of the Amen Clinics in America to have a brain scan which they specialise in. So far, I haven't been able to find anywhere that does the same in the UK or Europe and after learning about this I am so determined to have one. In short, they non-invasively scan the brain, as well as other assessments, to show the areas of the brain that are overactive, under active and/or not performing in the healthiest way. From this they can tailor a treatment plan that is most beneficial to you individually.

I can't explain how happy it makes me that with all of the support Jude has in place at such a young age, he won't have to struggle like I did, and will always have someone who understands him. The world is his oyster and I make sure he knows it.

The best way to predict the future is to create it.

Peter Drucker

Philosophical Author and Educator

Part Five

Advice And Information

HELPFUL TIPS FOR YOUR JOURNEY

Here are some things I have found helpful in coping throughout pre-diagnosis, learning, diagnosis, and post-diagnosis. This is advice I would have found helpful early on in my journey. I hope it can help you.

- First of all, start keeping a mood diary. At the end of every day write a few notes about how you have felt that day, anything you've struggled with, anything you've done well, how you slept etc. Keep this for a month or two.

- Spend some time researching the consistent issues/ struggles you're having –by consistent I mean as an example I knew something wasn't healthy about how I was feeling and behaving for years. It wasn't just difficult when I was dealing with particularly stressful things or when I wasn't sleeping well, it was also when

I 'should' have been at my happiest, when I had no other worries.

- For women, take note of any patterns from your mood diary with regards to your menstruation cycle and if it seems there is regularity with issues occurring at certain points, speak to your GP to ask for hormone and thyroid tests. Depending on your age it could be menopause-related which they should help with. Use your instinct as a guide to tell you that you are doing all you can and getting the help you deserve to feel better. Life does not have to be a struggle.

- If you feel you have a mental health issue, first of all, try the steps below with regards to diet, vitamins and general wellbeing. If this doesn't help or you are struggling significantly speak to your GP asap, they should be able to help you and if they don't seek advice from some of the contacts on the Recommended Resources section. Again, use your instinct as a guide to tell you that you are doing all you can and getting the help you deserve to feel better. Life does not have to be a struggle.

- If you believe that you could have ASC/ADHD, you will need to first speak with your GP. Please see the advice provided towards the end of the book.

- As I have previously mentioned if you do have ASC/ADHD, it is vital that you get an official assessment and diagnosis asap so that your treatment can start and that you begin to understand your mind, accept your diagnosis, and move forward positively.

- For ADHD there are medications available, both stimulants and non-stimulants as well as some antidepressant/anxiety medications. Most health professionals are not experienced enough to know the medications that will work for the different types of ADHD. I found it beneficial to take a test via Amen Clinics that I would recommend – www.theaddquiz.com. This free test will help you clarify the type of ADHD you have and advise you of the best treatment suitable for that type. For example, the right mix of medication for me is a stimulant and anxiety medication that enhances my serotonin and norepinephrine levels. You can also find this information in the book Healing ADD Revised Addition written by Dr Amen. Doing this will reduce the length of time it takes to find the most suitable treatment for you.

- Remember medication is not the first port of call; unless dealing with your issues is completely unbearable (as it was for me) then I would recommend trying the steps below regarding diet, vitamins, and general wellbeing before medication to see if they help first. You can always then try medication if you don't feel any better or if further down the line things become more difficult.

DIET AND VITAMINS

For most people with ASC/ADHD it is beneficial to eat a diet that is low in carbohydrates and high in protein. For all people, but especially those of us who are ND it is healthier for our brains to minimise sugar, dairy, wheat, processed meats and 'factory made' foods/snacks. Ideally, we should be eating organic food where possible. Alcohol and caffeine are particularly not good for those of us with ADHD and ASC if sleep is a struggle which it often is. Drinking plenty of water is also extremely important. You don't have to have a very restrictive diet (I can't as I love all foods) but you will figure out through making changes what works best and makes you feel good.

Vitamins can be highly beneficial for ND people and as a basic a 100% Multivitamin and 2000mg of Omega 3 Oil daily is good for our brains. The below are also known to be very helpful for those with ASC/ADHD and/or depression/anxiety:

WARNING – IF YOU TAKE ANY MEDICATIONS PLEASE CHECK WITH YOUR GP BEFORE TAKING

ANY OF THESE SUPPLEMENTS AS SOME CAN CAUSE
SERIOUS IMPLICATIONS IF USED TOGETHER

- Gingko Balboa
- Ashwaghanda
- 5HTP
- Vitamin D
- Vitamin B Complex
- Vitamin C
- Gaba
- Magnesium
- Evening Primrose Oil (for women)
- Probiotics
- Green Tea
- Rhodiola

GENERAL WELLBEING

Again, we should all be taking care of ourselves ND or
not, but in particular, if you have a brain that needs some
extra care, we need to do all we can to help it. A huge issue
to tackle when you have ASC/ADHD is sleep. We often
struggle to get to sleep, stay asleep and wake up when
needed. I have learned that setting an alarm to wake up
at the end of a sleep cycle works best for waking up. Sleep
cycles are around 1.5 hours, so for example if you go to sleep

at 11pm, six sleep cycles would take you to 8am. We need a minimum of 7.5 hours so tailor that to the time you have/want to wake up. Also try to stick to the same bedtimes and wake up times as much as possible so your body clock can get into a routine which is helpful. I have always loved my sleep and have been known to sleep for 16 hours if left alone and having had no alarm set (if I've been particularly tired); however, it isn't helpful for our mental health to sleep for this long so try and not go too far. If you do take medication, you will figure out what time is best for you to take it to help your sleep depending on your daily routine. Often people with ASC/ADHD struggle with restless legs at night in bed; I had suffered with this for a long time but finally found a high strength 100mg CBD oil that I take as I get into bed which honestly works miracles. Also, I don't drink for two hours before I go to bed, or at least not a big drink, so that I don't wake up to use the toilet because I would then struggle to get back to sleep.

Therapy can be so helpful for your mental health, especially if you have past issues that you need to work on. Past trauma can hugely affect our lives even if we're not aware of it or don't consciously think of it.

Regular exercise is well known to have massive benefits to those with ASC/ADHD and/or mental health issues. As I have mentioned, I am not a big fan of strenuous exercise such as running or going to the gym so I practise Pilates three times a week which I would recommend to anyone similar or anyone who has health issues that prevent them from doing too much physical exercise.

Lastly, daily routine is so important, consistency is such a benefit to all ND people. The self-care rituals that I have added to my daily routine have genuinely helped me live in a happier and more positive way. The book Manifest (details in Recommended Resources) teaches you the importance of listening to affirmations, repeating mantras, gratitude journalling, visualising and meditation to achieve a positive mindset. I cannot recommend these practices enough; they don't have to be for long periods – just 5-10 minutes can really calm our minds and give us peace.

As I tend to get tired later in the afternoon, I have learned to organise my days to get as much as possible done early in the day while I am focused and have more energy. I've also learned not to schedule too much into one day because it puts way too much pressure on me, and I then procrastinate and don't get anything done! I also space out any appointments as much as I can because one appointment literally takes up my whole day as I get anxious about having to be somewhere on time, and again, I will procrastinate. No matter how busy our lives are we must also always make time for ourselves, to rest, read a book, watch a movie, have a relaxing bath, give yourself a pamper treatment, just do nothing, or socialise – if you like to do that, some ND people, like me, don't.

Another thing which I have mentioned is how helpful it is to keep notes, to-do lists, things you want to discuss with someone or even just somewhere to write down the abundance of thoughts you may have so they're not just swirling around your mind overwhelming you. Also, I like to keep notes for when I have a bad day/s (which we ALL have) just to remind me that firstly, a bad day or a setback is not me relapsing into the awful state that I was in a few years ago! Then to write down what I am struggling with or worrying about and look at anything that I can change about my daily life etc to help. To communicate to my husband that I am overwhelmed and need space alone to sort things out and then to take that time to do that. To be kind to myself and remember that I simply cannot do it ALL – and that is true for everyone. To think logically about why I am feeling this way – is it lack of sleep or hormonal? Have there been any changes recently? Have I put pressure on myself to do too much? Lastly, to remind myself that ASC and ADHD are a part of who I am and that this will pass, and I will feel better again soon – experience has proven that.

It is a fact that you cannot love or care for others properly if you don't care for yourself, so treat yourself with kindness, treat yourself how you would your child or loved ones. Once you move into a more positive, healthy lifestyle and mindset you will automatically distance yourself from people or things that are negative for you, and you will learn what you really enjoy and what is best for you.

Lastly, I promise you can and will learn to love your brain for how it works and be grateful for the abilities it gives you in being different.

The challenge is
to be yourself in
a world where
everyone is trying
to make you be
somebody else.

E.E. Cummings

Poet, Author and Playwright

240

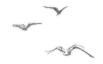

PARENTING A CHILD WITH ASC/ADHD

For ALL children having support, stability, routine, and love from the youngest age is proven to be essential to leading a happy life. For ND children this is even more important as it allows them to focus and work towards their potential and believing in themselves – knowing they are loved and understood unconditionally. As a society, we simply cannot complain about the increase in crime rates or levels of addiction, for example, without looking at how we can make positive change, and this all starts from childhood. If children are not nurtured and supported by their parents, wider family, school, government and health services, they quite simply cannot flourish as adults. The Princess of Wales recently launched a new campaign called Shaping Us, which is being hailed as "her life's work" and focuses on raising awareness of the vital role these early years play in shaping the rest of our lives. It is great to see a senior member of our Royal Family bringing attention to this and I truly hope that it will be highly beneficial for our children now and in the future.

To parents/carers of ND children:

The autistic children and children with ADHD of today, will in a few short years be autistic adults and adults with ADHD, and we need to give them as much support, love, confidence and understanding to allow them to achieve anything they want to in a world where they are accepted and needed. Please don't ever put them in a box, there is no limit to what ANYONE can achieve. Like any child, the hard work that we put in as parents will carry them through the rest of their lives. **PLEASE LET YOUR CHILD BE WHO THEY ARE.**

To parents/carers of ALL children:

We are all born pure, no hate, no discrimination, but children learn from their parents and the world around them – please don't forget the importance of teaching them to be kind and accept people for who they are. We're all different and that's a good thing, it's a necessary thing. We all want our children to grow up in a kind world.

In many areas, there is reluctance to diagnose children from a young age, which in my (and many others') opinion is wrong, as early intervention and support is vital and could be life changing – for the better. Not every child who is loud, shy, disruptive etc is ND, it could simply be their personality or a reflection of what they see at home; all behaviour is communication and if a child doesn't have boundaries, security and love they can act out in many ways. There are also many factors of the modern world that don't and can't cause ASC or ADHD, but they can cause similar behaviours. For example, the way in which many children depend on television, devices, and social media, and on the whole our society doesn't communicate in person like it used to. Also, a diet high in sugar and lacking in fresh food has a big impact. This will all be considered under their assessment.

I adore my son BUT parenting a child with ASC and/or ADHD how they need to be parented, is stressful, all-consuming and a lot of pressure. ALL parents are responsible for raising their children well enough for them to be happy, well-rounded people and when your child has additional needs it is us and only us who can get and give them the extra support, they need to achieve this. Since most grandparents in today's world are working longer than they did in the past, and our communities are more isolated, there is more pressure and less support for modern parents. I know it's overwhelming and daunting, but it really is only us who can do the job.

It can be hard being a parent to ANY child at times, for ANY mother or father – anyone who says it's easy is lying (or has a team of nannies). There are ways in which you can learn to support yourself on this journey as I have done. I would recommend for ND parents to make sure they schedule time for rest and self-care so that you don't burn out; this is essential, we can't be the best parents possible if we don't look after ourselves. For natural deep thinkers like myself the worry of having a child can be overwhelming; however, this is only because of the love I have for my child and again it's something I have learned to positively manage.

More than most other parents I know, I do struggle with leaving Jude in the care of others, partly because I want things exactly how they are at home for him and don't like the idea of not being fully in control of the way I know things work best for him. Jude being non-verbal obviously means it's difficult for others to communicate with him and him to them, and I do think some struggle with this. I worry when we're not there in the unlikely event of him feeling unwell or upset or angry, or just trying to communicate something, that it will be made worse for him by the fact that the person looking after him doesn't understand him. I never want Jude to feel like people don't understand him. All mums know our child best. Jude has an iPad device which is programmed with software to help him 'speak' so he can always request things such as food, or somewhere he wants to visit or family members etc. However, there are things such as his feelings or if he needs a break, that are hard to communicate using this. The older he gets the more he is trying to express himself as he is feeling all kinds of emotions and I am the best person to understand him and comfort him and stay calm in every situation. It's just intuitive and instinctive; other people can panic when they don't understand him which makes things worse. The only people who really 'get it' are other parents with ND children, and it is so helpful to connect with these people if we can and to keep learning.

With regards to Jude's speech issues, I came to see this as a blessing in disguise a long time ago now. If Jude hadn't been delayed with his speech, he would have more than likely gone undiagnosed which would have meant we wouldn't have been able to get him the support he needs so early in his life. I've met many families over the years whose children went under the radar but once they hit their teenage years the impact of living with ASC and/or ADHD without any help or intervention, greatly affects their behaviour, happiness, and wellbeing.

Also, as any parent of a child who has additional needs will know, it's truly special to be chosen for this path. We appreciate the smallest of things that other parents simply overlook as 'the norm', we celebrate every little milestone of development because we know what it has taken our children to get there. This makes life more exciting!

I want to clarify that we don't let Jude rule the roost and always do as he wishes, we also discipline him and push him out of his comfort zone. We don't let him have or do everything that he wants. Again, this is preparing him for the 'real world' because nobody gets what they want all of the time, and we explain this to him. We work with him on his communication and independence every day. He is the happiest boy you could meet and we're so proud of that, his smile lights up a room and his laugh is infectious. Like most parents I could go on forever about how special he is.

A lot of people wonder what it's like to be autistic and be a parent. I've read that some think autistic people won't make good parents because they're selfish and couldn't look after a child. Well, this is completely false – I for one am obsessed with my son, and my neurodivergent ability to learn about subjects important to and for him, has undoubtedly helped him so far in life. That will continue to be the case until he finds his voice and becomes independent (and probably still then, let's be honest). I understand him and I can relate to him in a way that others cannot. Also, some of the ways in which we need to help Jude come easily for me as it is part of me too, for example, routine and repetitiveness.

Lastly, I want to share a positive story that I hope will bring you hope if/when needed – I have read many similar stories over the years that always positively support my vision for Jude – and whilst writing, the below was shared in the media:

Jason Arday of London, England, was diagnosed with autism aged three years old and was non-verbal until age eleven. He learned how to read and write aged eighteen. Currently, at age thirty-seven, Jason has become the youngest black person ever to be appointed a professorship at Cambridge University.

If Jason (and many others around the world) can do it, so can your child.

It is easier to build strong children than to repair broken men

Frederick Douglass

Historical Civil Rights Leader

ADVICE FOR PARENTS OF A CHILD WITH ASC/ADHD

- Trust your instinct. You know your child better than anyone.

- If you suspect they have ASC or ADHD, seek a referral for assessment and don't give up until you have them assessed.

- Make notes of all the reasons why you think they have ASC/ADHD as sometimes in the assessment process children's true behaviour isn't shown (particularly in girls) and you may forget their issues/needs when asked on the spot, so it can be helpful to keep a diary beforehand.

- If needed, remember getting a diagnosis is of benefit to your child because without it they will not receive the support they need, particularly in education. It has nothing to do with your opinion or preconceived ideas of either condition. BEING ND IS NOT A NEGATIVE.

- If your child is autistic and/or has ADHD, the longer they go without understanding themselves, and receiving the right support, the harder life will be for them in the future. I have met so many parents over the years who put it off, but issues ALWAYS arise at some point and then it can be too late to really help them. Early intervention is so important to allow them to live happily and to reach their potential.

- Taking advice or looking at other people's experiences online can be helpful but don't take everything you read as gospel. Remember everyone is different and only a medical professional can diagnose your child. Make your own opinions and don't be scared by what other people think about ASC and/or ADHD. Stay away from negativity, nothing good comes from it. See Recommended Resources pages for some safe sites.

- Don't be in denial about any issues your child may have. We all think our children are perfect, and they are, but that doesn't mean they don't need support in some areas. Pretending it isn't happening DOES NOT help them in any way.

- Read the books and watch the films/shows I have recommended. Even though you may not feel like they apply to your child or that your child is different to them, it is still valuable knowledge.

- Read positive stories about children with ASC and/or ADHD to give you the hope and strength that you may need to keep going with the work you do.

- There is nothing that unconditional love and support cannot help, and I have seen it with my own eyes from many other ND families and ND adults who have achieved so much more than what 'professionals' or opinions estimated. Nobody KNOWS FOR SURE what ANYONE is or isn't capable of in the right environment.

- Stay positive and optimistic, nobody knows what the future holds and what advances in care, support and knowledge will have been made in another 10-20 plus years.

- Remember your child is special. Every child is special but people with ASC and/or ADHD are in the minority and have a truly individual way of thinking and behaving. An autistic child will leave everyone wanting more of them once they start to communicate/interact with them because it is a privilege for them to notice you and their affection is pure and honest – if they love you it's genuine.

- Connect with other parents of children with ASC and/or ADHD to communicate and share the journey with. Nobody understands like another ND family. You can ask your child's school or health visitor etc to put you in touch with other parents and your local council will most likely have details of SEN groups.

- Fully believe that your child can do ANYTHING with your love and support because they can, and let them know this, so they believe it themselves. Do not put them in a box and write off their potential because they are ND.

- Remember EVERYONE learns at different times and in different ways so NEVER compare your child to others.

- NEVER give up on your child. When it seems impossible, take a break, reassess, and move forward. Remember they can't advocate for themselves yet.

- Enjoy your child for who they are. It may be different to what you expected but childhood goes so fast so don't waste it by worrying about the next milestone they're going to reach, for example, or whatever stage it is you wish they were at.

- Focus on what they CAN do, not what they CANNOT do, YET.

- Teach your child that their brain works differently and how that is a gift, this way they won't grow up confused about why they feel different to others and that they will be confident that it's not a bad thing to be different.

- As difficult as it is, try and make time for yourself when you can, it makes you a better parent. ASK for help if you need it.

- Fight to get them into the right school, or for the best education plan for them, whether it's mainstream, SEN or private, it doesn't matter if it's right for them and YOU WILL KNOW.

- Have a good working relationship with your child's school, SLT, paediatrician, OT and any other professionals that work with them. Let them know you are involved and that any advice that you can get, you want. Ask them if there are things you can be doing at home to help your child or if there is any other help you think they would benefit from. Let them know that if there is any training available you would like to attend and keep doing this throughout your child's journey because things change all the time as your child grows.

- Also schedule regular reviews with your child's teacher, and the other staff that work with them in school, to make sure that you're all on the same page and that your child is happy and moving forward, working towards their potential. Again, if you don't arrange this yourself it most likely won't get done as school staff are extremely busy and have many other children to look after – you just have yours.

- Also, if your child has an EHCP this will be reviewed annually so make a note of this in your diary/calendar and proactively make sure that it is arranged on time. In 12 months, children change and progress A LOT so everyone involved with your child needs to be aware of the current and future targets etc, and you need to make sure the support they can get is up to date or amended if necessary.

- If your child is struggling to toilet train, ask for a referral to your local continence team – you'll be amazed at how things can change literally overnight when you put the effort in, and when something just 'clicks'. This was one of the biggest challenges for us: Jude literally went from pooping on the living room carpet and playing with it one day, with no understanding whatsoever, to taking himself off to the toilet and having no accidents ever again the next.

- Sign up for your local authority's SEN newsletter, which will include free parent training courses and local activities for your family.

- If your child is non-verbal or has limited speech, use the Hanen techniques at home. Read the book I have recommended, and this will teach you everything you can do at home to help your child communicate. The most important thing is firstly to find a way for them to tell you their basic needs such as hunger, thirst, toilet etc.

- If your child is non-verbal, or has limited speech, look at funding for devices to help them communicate.

- Remember all behaviour is communication, so if your child is unhappy, angry, or frustrated etc, help them show you to figure out why. Do they need more ways to communicate? Do they need down time? Do they need to release some energy? You will soon come to understand what it is they're saying even if it's not in speech.

- Our children, especially if limited in communication, can be more vulnerable than other children, sadly; for this reason I never tell Jude to do as he's told (unless he's with me) because you never know how literally they will take this and think that they have to do everything EVERY grown up tells them. I also tell him that if anyone or anything ever upsets him or hurts him, to tell me, show me a picture I will understand.

- Let your child know each day what their plans are for the day. I repeat this several times through the day and use now and next pictures. Prepare them as much as you can and explain everything you're doing as much as possible. This isn't just for the importance of their routine but also because children learn language from us.

- Teach them to have fun, try their best and not to worry. I explain to Jude that we all have different feelings sometimes, but that we will always be happy again soon so not to worry. Autistic children can struggle to express themselves, so I like Jude to understand, and be open about, his feelings.

- Always remember your child is listening and can understand every word you say, even if they look like they're in another world. IT IS GOING IN ALL THE TIME. Don't talk about them like they're not there or talk negatively about them or their condition.

- We have always 'pushed' Jude into doing things outside of his comfort zone as that is how you learn, grow, and overcome certain things. However, do not push your child, especially one with limited communication, into doing anything that they clearly are super anxious or fearful of. For example, when Jude started at school, he was invited to a lot of birthday parties and he loves going to soft play or trampoline parks etc. However, there was one party held in a small church hall with a DJ and kids' entertainers and it was LOUD. There was not much space, and it was just completely overwhelming. He took one look inside and was terrified, which isn't like him at all, so we didn't make him go in. Other than being alongside the children, which he was often anyway, there was no real benefit for him going in and as I've said we have to choose our battles – this really wasn't important. We consoled him, told him he was safe and that it was no big deal, and we took him to the park which he loves. It didn't need to be a negative experience/memory and he knew we understood him and felt safe.

- Like every other parent/child you will know what they like, what they don't, when they're just being spoilt or when they NEED or CANNOT do something. When they need quiet time, the phases they go through – be confident in that and know that you will instinctively always do your best for them. Not everything they do is because they are autistic or have ADHD, so bear that in mind and don't treat them differently to other children where possible.

- Regardless of whether your child is verbal, partially verbal, or non-verbal, children often can't express themselves very well. Like all parents we get to know our child and their behaviours inside out, so remember to follow their cues for things they need such as quiet time. We all need time alone and peace and quiet, so if your child doesn't want to engage 24/7, don't make them as that is pointless. If they get the downtime they need, they will be more willing to engage afterwards. It is more than ok to give them a break and to give yourself one too.

- Another example regarding this is that Jude is very rarely ill or upset so as he cannot verbally tell me that he doesn't feel well I have learned that if he is emotional or cries for no obvious reason along with looking pale and not wanting to eat, then he isn't feeling good, and I can then take care of him in the necessary way. We also ask Jude to show us what is hurting, if we know he has had a little fall, for example, and he will point to the part of his body that is hurting.

- Expose them to socialising as much as possible from as young as possible – the more they're around other people the more they will get used to it and accept it. They may still like to play alone but that's ok, let them do what they are comfortable doing if it isn't harming anyone.

- If you don't have much of a social circle then make sure your child goes to a playgroup, nursery, or pre-school to get used to being around their peers from a young age.

- Take them out and about with you as much as possible from as young as possible. Being sheltered is not beneficial to the rest of their life. Also try to take them swimming regularly if you can, as being in the water is proven to be therapeutic for ND children – you can physically see them calm down when they're submerged.

- We have practised vestibular and proprioceptive exercises with Jude since he was three years old, you can find many examples online to do at home. They are proven to help with brain development and are also a calming tool for our children who often need to feel deep muscle pressure.

- It is great if you can arrange play dates with other children on the spectrum and/or with ADHD. They may not play TOGETHER but being around other children with similar needs to themselves, gives them confidence and takes the pressure off. They may not even seem like they notice or are indifferent to it, but they WILL be taking it in.

- Comfortable, loose clothing is generally preferable to autistic children/people, so try to remove any tags or labels prior to them wearing anything. Don't worry about putting them in jeans and a fancy shirt to go to a play centre, maybe save these outfits for special occasions and even then, only ask them to wear it if they're happy to, allow them to be as free and at ease as possible as they already have so many heightened sensory feelings.

- Explain any changes in routine, or for example if you have a holiday coming up, by using visual aids/pictures, if necessary, in as far advance as possible.

- If there are events coming up such as a parent going into hospital you can buy Social Stories online which will help you explain things in a way they will understand.

- Try not to worry about how your child will take to different things, it is often more our own worry than the child's. Just give it a chance.

- Allow friends/family to spend time with your child and get to know them well so that you have the possibility of respite as this is very important, it's also good for your child to develop relationships with other people and not to be completely dependent on you.

- If someone else is looking after your child, don't be worried about seeming overprepared when you want to set up the bedroom for them or want to give them a long list of things to do and not to do, and/or a routine. Ask them what their plans are and advise them what is best for your child in different situations. Always be contactable as you could quickly diffuse a difficult situation for your child as you know them best and will understand what their problem is.

- Make sure you tell EVERYONE who works with, or spends time with, your child, about their needs/communication/issues/behaviours, so they can work with you on being the best for your child. Don't be afraid to give information or tell people about any diagnosis. Most people who work with children and/or who have only just met them will find it super helpful to have this information. Again, it is up to us to speak up for what our child needs.

- Keep trying because things change – for example, if your child has never wanted to eat vegetables this doesn't mean they never will. Don't make a big issue out of small things, you will quickly learn to choose your battles – does it really matter if they don't eat every fruit/vegetable or aren't very adventurous with food if they are healthy and getting their needs met in some way?

- Enjoy your child, even watching them play or being in their own world, and show interest in whatever it is that your child is interested in – they may not want you to join in what they're doing but showing them that you are interested in them, and their interests is so beneficial for building connections.

- Jude is currently non-verbal, but his communication has progressed massively in the last few years, I believe because we have consistently implemented many things at home that we have learned over this time. I won't go in to too much detail as I do recommend the book later, but a book from Hanen pretty much taught us everything in the early days. For example, when Jude was three years old, we took and printed out photos of all the things he used at home. Items such as his drink cup, foods, toilet, television, garden and pictures of us and all our family members, and we have these freely available in their own place at home for whenever he would like to use them – of course they have been updated over the years as he has grown. The first day we did this he came to us in the morning when he woke up with a picture of his cup for his milk – that was first time he had been able to communicate a request or need to us, and it was amazing! Something so simple but hugely beneficial for us all.

- We keep our words simple when talking directly to Jude, when asking him a question or giving him an instruction, so he can understand and learn the words more easily. At first making these changes may seem overwhelming but trust me when I say it's worth it and it becomes second nature after a while – every child I speak to now I speak to in this same way without thinking.

- Talk to them about anything, as much as you can. They are always listening and soaking in everything you say and how you behave. Reading to your child is also proven to help bonding and communication so if you're ND yourself and talking constantly isn't for you, then reading is a way in which you can communicate.

- Repeat, repeat, repeat everything and anything you say and do. This is how we all learn both communication and physical activities such as getting dressed or washing, through repetition.

- The main areas we can benefit our child's lives, are total belief in them, showing them they are supported and secure, giving them a routine, set them boundaries, and helping them live a healthy life with food and exercise, from infancy.

- Diarise dates to chase up any referrals or assessments your child has been sent for because if you don't nobody will magically do it for you. It shouldn't be the case, but those who advocate the loudest and the most, often do benefit.

- We speak about autism and ADHD openly with and around Jude (not in an overwhelming way as he is still young) because we never want it to be a secret or for them to be negative subjects.

- As Jude gets older, I am exposing him to as many different activities and interests as possible so that he can find what his passions in life are and we will then support him with those.

- Something I find difficult, but know I MUST do, is allow Jude to be independent as much as possible. As he is an only child I do like to 'mother' him quite a lot, but I do make myself (I also tell others including school to do the same) let him do things for himself such as getting dressed even if it takes a while, wash himself, open his drinks bottle, wipe his bum and wash his hands, feed himself and put his shoes on etc. Autistic children may take a bit longer to learn (and be physically able to do such things due to the lack of motor skills the condition can carry), but they can be more than capable of doing them with support and patience. Not everything a ND child does is down to their ND, like EVERY other child, they can just be being lazy or pushing the boundaries.

- For many reasons, other typical milestones may take longer than a NT child to learn, but again this is fine, and they should feel NO PRESSURE. For example, toilet training, night-time toilet training, riding a bike, talking at the same level as their peers, using a knife and fork, self-hygiene and reading and writing. There is no rush, they have a lifetime of being adults.

- Autistic children, like ALL children, go through phases, so remember this if things get particularly difficult: it will pass.

- If the work is put in early and support is available, our children CAN and DO, do anything. For whatever reasons, some say it's because their brains are so occupied with other things, for example, things can take longer to connect in their ND brains, but they will, and it doesn't matter at what point this is.

- If you possibly can, allow your child to have a room or space at home that is their quiet space where they can go and relax and be alone safely. Ideally it needs to be clutter-free, quiet, soothing so not too bright or colourful, grey is a good colour, a weighted blanket, and a beanbag to lie on for example, and allow them to take their iPad/games/toys/books or similar in there for some real relaxing downtime, as it is much needed.

- Again, if you can (also you can always ask friends and family to help when it's Christmas or a birthday) get them some sensory toys and equipment for at home and your garden if you have one. Keep some at any other homes your child may visit too as this is really helpful. For example, fidget toys, squeezy toys, stretchy toys, trampolines, climbing frames, weighted vests, swings, peanut balls, and exercise balls.

- Jude has had the same bedtime routine since he was born; his bedroom is all grey with no toys or other distractions. There is no lightbulb in the light fitting so he can't turn it on at 3am. He has a soft lamp for when we do his bedtime story. Also, his bedding and pyjamas are always fresh, soft, and comfortable. These are just some of the ways in which you can help the quality of your child's sleep which they will inevitably struggle with at some points in their life due to their condition. Sleep is so, so important to health, both physical and mental, and they NEED to rest their growing minds and bodies which are very active.

- ANYONE professional you speak to regarding your child during this journey, whether it's someone at your local authority, child development centre, hospital, school, SLT or OT etc, take their name and number. Half of the battle with getting anywhere is having someone to contact directly or different people in the same office telling you different things. Build a relationship or connection with anyone you can as this will help your child hugely even years down the line.

- As hard as it may seem, don't worry about your child's future or what they will and won't be able to do that you thought they would or that other children of their age will be doing. Nowadays what is a 'normal' life? For example, not everyone wants to have a family, get married, have a partner, have a 9-5 job, work until they're 65 and then retire. Times have changed and we should only encourage our children to do what makes THEM happy, not us and not anyone else. The goals that NT people have for their futures and happiness aren't necessarily the same as what ND people want. Being popular, being rich or living independently, for example, often don't matter if we are getting enjoyment from our own interests. NT people don't generally need or want to have a special interest that they enjoy but for us ND people it brings us comfort and self-worth to have a passion.

- Lastly, be grateful that your child is here, is healthy and learn to relax and enjoy them for who they are. You might be daunted that you may have to support them into adulthood, but really, ALL parents do this anyway, at least good ones, we don't wash our hands of them the minute they turn 18 and say job done. They will need us for the rest of our lives.

- There are parents, with grown up children who have late diagnoses, who feel terribly guilty for not noticing the signs that their child was ND or struggling in their younger years. Please DO NOT feel this way, no good can come from it for either of you. Even just a few years ago, ASC and ADHD were nowhere near as highlighted as they are now, and without the information, there is no possible way you could have known. Remember NOW there IS an abundance of information and guidance which you can use to support your child. For those with children who are still young, it is our job to prepare our

ND kids for their future. It would have been SO helpful had I known many years ago what ND was, how my brain works, how there is nothing 'wrong' with me and the ways in which to manage the conditions earlier.

Jude's Daily Routine Basics

1. Jude will have his breakfast (gluten-free cereal similar to Weetabix, with fruit blended in) and take his multivitamin and Omega 3 oil capsules.

2. His pictures for the day will be on the dining table for him and we will discuss his plans and tell him who is picking him up from school.

3. School

4. After school we will often go to the park or to visit family.

5. I will always let Jude know his plans for the rest of the day.

6. When we get home Jude will have a snack, usually fruit, and then we will do some vestibular and proprioceptive exercises and massage. During this time, I will chat to Jude about his day and discuss any upcoming plans etc.

7. I will read to Jude before he has some downtime with his iPad.

8. Around two hours before bedtime, the television and Jude's iPad are turned off and any lights turned down. We play some calming music and Jude has no drinks from now (except a very small one after dinner).

9. We have dinner and Jude's pictures for the next day will be on the dining table. After dinner Jude has his night-time vitamins (magnesium and calcium).

10. Bath time and then one of us gives Jude a calming massage and we read the same quick bedtime story before going to sleep.

A child seldom needs a good talking to as much as a good listening to

Robert Brault

Inspirational Writer

COMMON TRAITS OF ASC (AND HOW THEY CAN BE SUPPORTED)

Please remember that those with ASC have varying behaviours, skills, and personalities just like everyone else in the world. It is a huge spectrum and having some of the below traits alone does not make you autistic and not all autistic people have the same traits; also, an autistic person won't necessarily have to have all of these traits. Being autistic affects each individual differently.

In children:

- **Avoids or does not keep eye contact** – Once you are aware of this you can practise reminding your child to look at people in the eye; however, I don't think it's detrimental if this doesn't feel comfortable, do you? I personally learned to do this by watching other people around me and knowing it was expected, but it has never felt comfortable, and I have always had to force myself to do it. It's a learned behaviour now but I try and not force myself anymore.

- **Does not respond to name** – This will come with time and routine, don't stop using your child's name or speaking to them in general, because you think they don't understand, because they do, and the more they hear words the more they will.

- **Does not show facial expression** – You can overly express your feelings on your face so that in time your child gets used to what this means and may pick it up. Also verbalise what each emotion you're showing is – such as sad for a cry, happy for a smile and anger for a frown. They will also work on emotions in school.

- **Does not imitate actions/gestures such as clapping hands or waving** – This will come with time and practice, but again I always think it's not a big deal and not something we HAVE to make children do. Often the child knows exactly HOW to do it, they just don't WANT to.

- **Does not participate in simple interactive games** – This takes a lot of practice and school will help, but at the end of the day some people just don't like to play/interact in the same way as other people. You can practise at home; it helps to use motivating toys/games to keep them interested – you can search for these easily online. Also, using a reward system is helpful, as are 'now and next' pictures.

- **Does not share interests with others** – This will come with time and experience. Keep sharing your interests with them, you can guarantee that in school or social settings other children will be happy to share theirs and hopefully in the future your child will be interested in sharing their own. You will also work out what their interests are by watching them and seeing what they gravitate towards or enjoy doing, and once you do it is very helpful to join them (if they allow you) or to at least positively comment on what they're interested in to show them you're also interested.

- **No or limited speech by age two years** – Working with a SLT (Speech Language Therapist) will help. You can do a lot of work at home such as using simple language and visual aids (again please refer to my recommendation of the Hanen book). There is a lot of technology that can be used now, which again is something that will only improve with time. Your child will find a way to communicate, you just have to do your research and find the best support and schooling. This is why getting a diagnosis is so important because you will have access to much more support once this is in place.

- **Does not show you things by pointing** – This will come with time but again it's something that I never thought was a big deal. Many autistic children struggle with their fine motor skills (for example it can take them several years to be able to correctly hold a pencil), but with practice and exercises their muscles will get stronger and they will be able to do more with their hands, it just takes them a little longer to catch up.

- **Seems not to notice other children or join them in play** – As I've already explained, often autistic children like to be around other children even if it doesn't seem like it, so don't isolate them, and remember to make things as comfortable as possible for them to enjoy the experience. Most autistic children are more than happy to play 'alongside' others but not necessarily 'with them', which is fine. School will help in this area and just try to make it a common occurrence, so they get used to it and feel at ease and therefore more likely to relax and be themselves which is the most important thing.

- **Does not play imaginatively, for example pretending to be a teacher** – Being at school/nursery and around other children of all abilities will help but some children just don't like to play like others may do. I wasn't a big role player and even now that's my husband's department with Jude or our nieces and nephew, because it just doesn't feel natural to me.

- **Has repetitive behaviours such as lining up toys** – Don't stop your child doing this, even if you think it looks a bit strange. Let them continue if it makes them happy and isn't dangerous. This is a form of 'stimming', and it causes no harm, and unless it becomes obsessive it's an activity that helps them stay calm and regulated. Stimming, short for self-stimulatory behaviour, is the repetition of either physical movements, sounds, words or objects and it regulates stress and other emotions and can also help with sensory input. ALL of us 'stim' at some level (for example tapping your foot, biting your nails, or twirling your hair around your finger), we just don't notice it. Some 'stimming' behaviours are more 'socially acceptable' than others, but that doesn't make them better, just more common.

- **Flaps hands, spins, rocks their body, and climbs everything in sight** – As above these actions are more forms of stimming and should not be viewed as a negative behaviour or stopped, unless maybe you are somewhere where it is inappropriate or it is causing harm. If this is the case explain that to the child and they will learn with time. Often, autistic older children/ adults learn to do this in their own home where they are more understood and comfortable as they learn how to manage their behaviours and where certain things are and aren't appropriate. For example, Jude went through a stage of banging on everything he could see; he was looking for deep sensory stimulus. This was fine on the carpet at home or even the walls, we didn't mind and understood, but he quickly had to learn that he couldn't walk around the shops and bang on shelves and cash desks as this is not acceptable behaviour and can be disruptive. I explained that he could do certain things at home that we can't when we're out or in other people's homes etc. Also, OT support can help if stimming becomes disruptive or harmful.

- **Focuses on only the same part of a toy such as spinning the wheels on a car** – This is another stimming behaviour, and I would advise as above.

- **Has obsessive interests** – if the obsession is becoming inappropriate, unhealthy, or having a negative effect on their daily life or others, then an OT can help; however, it's ok for people to have their own hobbies and interests even if they are a little different. It can be surprising what needs are being met by the things our children do, for example, my son had a habit of constantly clapping, which sounds harmless enough, but he has a very loud clap, and I was worried his hands would get sore and it was almost like he was being controlled by the need to clap. We spoke to the OT at his school and discovered this was a way for Jude to get deep muscle pressure that he needed, so they changed his sensory diet in school, and he swims every morning now which helps massively, and we got him a weighted vest to wear if needed and some compression leggings to wear at home, and we do a lot of deep pressure massage at home and the clap phase passed!

- **Gets upset by minor changes** – We all need to learn that change is inevitable whether we like it or not, but at least while they're young and still learning, try to keep change to a minimum and if it is unavoidable try to explain this to the child, giving them as much notice as possible. It's helpful to use visual aids such as pictures to show them the plan, what is happening 'now and next'. Repetition is key for people with ASC so repeat the plans as many times as possible to help them take it in. For an example, I was recently taking a trip with my sister for six nights, which is by far the most time I have ever left Jude for. The week before I created an

A4 laminated chart showing the days of the week and had small passport size photos printed of everyone who would be helping with Jude while I was away and then a picture of me on the day I was coming home. He was shown this every day and it was left out for him to look at.

- **Unusual sleeping patterns** – This can be one of the hardest areas of parenting a child with ASC and it's a vicious circle because children need sleep to develop and sustain attention and the less sleep they get the harder it is. We all NEED sleep, it's vital, it's helpful to follow a strict bedtime routine such as lights down and low volume around two hours before, no TV or iPad etc two hours before, no drinks an hour or so before, or if necessary just sips, try not to send them to bed hungry but not too full either, no sugar several hours before, a comfortable bed with sensory-aware bedding and pyjamas, a warm bath, lavender oil – not too much – and deep pressure massage on their joints as they lie in bed. Keep things short and sweet when you leave the room. If a child is very upset or afraid, my advice would be to do what is best for your whole family to get sleep – it won't last forever. Also, if necessary, you can speak to your child development centre who can help with advice and support or medication. Don't suffer in silence.

- **Unusual eating habits** – Try as best you can to encourage your child to eat with you at mealtimes and to eat a varied diet. This really needs to start from when they begin weaning as a baby to get them used to it. They need to experience all different textures and temperatures of food. Also, time and experience will allow their palates and confidence in trying new things to grow. You can try blending fruit and vegetables into their meals so they're not aware they're there. Jude has always loved fruit and veg pouches (like smoothies) which was good when he wasn't as adventurous at a younger age, but he still likes them now. However, the fact is, mainly due to sensory issues, some autistic children (and adults) genuinely find it impossible to eat anything other than a few basic items. You will need professional help with this as their diet is so important for their health and development. If they are missing out on vitamins there are many ways you can get them into their digestive system, such as through hiding multivitamin liquids in drinks or yogurt, or using vitamin gummies that look like sweets. Omega 3 Oil is particularly beneficial to ND children and adults. Contact your health visitor or child development centre if this becomes a real problem beyond general childhood fussiness. However, as I have already mentioned, not every behaviour is because of ND. EVERY child can be fussy with food so remember this when you are disciplining them or don't know what way to go with it – you will know your child best.

- **Lack of fear** – this will come with time but use any opportunity to explain dangers to them and don't overlook the fact that you need to be always with them when near traffic etc, and in car parks. What may be common sense to you doesn't mean the same for them. As with anything you're trying to teach your child, repeating yourself is key to them taking it in.

- **Gastrointestinal issues such as constipation** – Many children with ASC struggle with this and there are solutions that can be prescribed by your GP to help soften their stools. Half the problem can be that the child is scared to go to the toilet because it hurts. Try and have them drink as many fluids as possible throughout the day, and fruit and vegetables help. If they don't like eating fruit and vegetables, you can try organic smoothie pouches as it has the same effect, but autistic children seem to prefer the texture etc. Contact your GP with these issues and, if necessary, they can refer you to your local continence team.

In older children/adults:

- **Finds joining in a conversation difficult OR can dominate a conversation OR talks AT people rather than TO people** – Being around understanding people makes this less of a problem; obviously it's not ideal to come across as rude, but awareness of these behaviours and the wish to learn and grow will come with age, time, and experience. It may be helpful to practise at home.

- **Uses repetitive language** – This can be a habit and, in my opinion, not too much of a problem unless it's inappropriate, which an SLT can help with.

- **Has trouble reading social cues** – This comes with time, practice, experience, and support from those around you.

- **Takes things literally** – This may always be the case; it can be a humorous side of our personality and gets easier with age and experience.

- **Can be blunt in their assessment of people or things** – Of course, it's never ok to be mean and we ALL need to learn that, again we need to learn what is or isn't appropriate and we can do so with support from those around us, education, experience, and time.

- **Others find it hard to know how they are feeling** – This can be hard, and I know that people find me difficult to read; however, with time the people around you will learn to understand you and you can practise how to express yourself to others if you would like to.

- **Finds it difficult to maintain eye contact** - I personally feel uncomfortable doing this, but I have learned with time that in some cases it's appropriate, so I do, and it comes as second nature now although it doesn't feel natural to me. I don't think it's a huge deal if it is comfortable for you and those around you will understand you. If you want to you can teach yourself to do this with time and practice.

- **Anxious in social situations** - Having understanding people around you and family, therapy, and the willingness to come out of your comfort zone to do things you enjoy can help with this. Don't push yourself too much if it's not something you want to do, but if you do it can become easier.

- **Finds it hard to express themselves** - This can come with time, practice, and support; it helps to read about the subject and therapy is good to help you understand your emotions/feelings.

- **Can invade people's space** - Obviously, this is usually not appropriate and while family and friends may not mind, others most likely will, so practise with family members, and help from an OT and education providers can assist too.

- **Speaks in a monotone voice** – We all have different voices and that's fine. If you want to add more 'personality' to your voice you can practise if you wish, which can help you build a habit of controlling how you speak, much like elocution lessons. SLT support can also help with this if necessary.

- **Finds building and maintaining close friendships difficult** – This is something that takes time and effort from both sides, so it helps to choose friends who are kind, understanding people. Also be honest about your condition with new people you meet, which should help them understand you more. Therapy can also help, along with support from those around you, and experience.

- **Has trouble regulating emotional responses** – This comes with time, and it helps to read lots about this subject; also, therapy is good to help you understand your emotions/feelings and how to manage them.

- **Does not like their things being moved by anyone else** – Make the people around you aware of how this makes you feel, and they should accept your wishes; they may not be aware of how it makes you feel so need to be told.

- **Notices small details, smells, or patterns that others don't** – This can be a wonderful quality to have and is why so many people with ASC excel in their chosen area of work/hobby. If it becomes obsessive, an OT and/or therapy can help. It can also be a hindrance because as our senses are heightened, we might smell or hear things that we don't want to, but we can learn to manage this with time.

- **Has very strong reactions to sensory stimulation such as smells, noises, and textures** – There are so many different stimuli that can overwhelm BUT there is a lot of advice online to help manage this more comfortably plus OT support can help. However, in my experience the main areas are sound – so be aware of the volume in which the person is comfortable and wearing headphones can help; smell – strong smells such as perfume and certain foods can be a problem so try to bear this in mind and allow as much fresh air as possible; textures – labels on clothes often need to be cut out to feel comfortable, the texture of foods are often the issue with fussy eaters rather than the taste and slimy or messy textures are usually not ideal to touch – in general, we don't like being messy!

- **Must follow routines** – This can be another method of stimming which can worsen at times of stress. Keeping to a routine makes us feel comfortable and allows us to have some order when we are overwhelmed. Unless it negatively affects your daily life, in which case therapy or OT support can help, this is a part of you and can be a positive. Personally, I thrive off routine.

- **Can become upset if their schedule changes** – Routine can be good for everyone and as explained above it can be a self-stimulatory behaviour for those with ASC; however, change is inevitable in life, and it takes time to learn how to accept change, even if it doesn't feel great. The more we experience this, the easier it gets and repetitive explanations in advance help a lot.

- **Has repetitive rituals that they follow daily** – This is just a part of who we are and helps keeps us calm as it can also be self-stimulatory behaviour, and as long as it isn't hurting anyone there shouldn't be an issue. If it becomes obsessive or interrupts daily life, an OT and/ or therapy can help. Again, it can very much be part of a need to have an order when we're overwhelmed, which helps us greatly. Other stimming behaviours can include frequent blinking, clearing throat repeatedly, turning head side to side, repeating the same song, tapping, or flicking fingers, clenching fists, grinding teeth, and rubbing hands together.

- **Has difficulty multitasking** – This can improve with time and practice and sometimes it just is what it is, but if it becomes a real problem in daily life OT support can help.

- **Has an object or area of specific interest that they spend a lot of time on** – This can be a great talent! However, if the obsession becomes inappropriate or is having a negative effect on your daily life then support from an OT can help. But, REMEMBER it's ok for people to have their own hobbies and interests even if they are a little different to the 'norm'.

- **Struggles with anxiety and/or depression** – This is highly likely at times for those with ASC simply because it can be overwhelming and without awareness and support can feel unmanageable. Therapy is extremely helpful as can be medication, and general advice for mental health is applicable, as well as an understanding about your condition/s. Please refer to the Helpful Tips section.

- **Walks on tiptoes –** This is very common and can be done for many reasons, such as stimming, and the person having balance or co-ordination issues. Usually, we grow out of this in time, but if not and/or it becomes a real problem then OT support can help.

- **Struggles with body posture and/or walks 'funny'** – Many of us with ASC suffer with our joints and hypermobility which means we can appear to have an 'unusual' gait or struggle to hold ourselves 'correctly'. Many of us also feel more comfortable sitting on the floor rather than a chair. We can practise using the 'correct' posture at home and there are support braces that can also help. Again, support from an OT can help.

- **Rigid thinking** – Like any of our traits we do not choose to be difficult of think rigidly; it is the way our brain works. For example, it is not easy for us to change tasks, we can struggle to think or concentrate on anything else than our hyper focused interest/s, we struggle with change in routine, especially when stressed or tired, and this may make it look like we are rigid in our thinking. We need those around us to understand this and to accept us for who we are in a positive light.

- **May struggle with using a knife and fork or holding a pen** – Many autistic people have low muscle tone; we don't know why but it's just another (so far) unexplained issue that comes with our condition. This can affect our fine motor skills BUT over time and with practice we can and do pick up these skills; it just may take a while longer than those who are NT.

COMMON TRAITS OF ADHD (AND HOW THEY CAN BE SUPPORTED)

Please remember that those with ADHD have varying behaviours, skills, and personalities just like everyone else in the world. Having some of the below traits alone does not mean you have ADHD and not all people with ADHD have the same traits; also, a person with ADHD won't necessarily have all of these traits. Having ADHD affects each individual differently.

In children:

- **Short attention span** – Over time this should naturally improve as the child gets older –, a lot of NT children have limited attention too. However, it is helpful to work on this at home and find individual ways to help. Medication can also help greatly with this if it continues to be an issue affecting daily life. We also need to make sue our children are in the best school setting for the needs which will help.

- **Easily distracted** – Again, this is something many NT children also struggle with, and it can be something that they grow out of, but again individual practice and medication can help if it continues and starts to affect their daily life. We also need to make sure our children are in the best school setting for the needs which will help.

- **Makes careless mistakes** – As their attention/concentration improves with age this should help; however, my advice would be to try not to force a child with ADHD to do things they have no interest in because it will be almost impossible for them to take in and they CAN excel in areas they are interested in!

- **Appears forgetful or often loses things** – Firstly, try not to be frustrated with the child or at least try not to show them that you are. It will be just as frustrating to them if not more so and they don't need that pressure. You can teach them to write things down that they need to remember and to have specific places for important items, so they don't lose them. Routine also helps a lot.

- **Appears unable to listen and carry out instructions** – Try to give instructions or important information when the child is engaged. Ask them to write down what you have asked them to do to help them remember.

- **Constantly changing activity** – If it's not hurting anyone, in my opinion, this is quite harmless. All children need to try many different activities to find out what they're interested in and what their passions are, so exposing them to as many different areas as possible is a good thing.

- **Difficulty organising tasks** – Writing things down helps massively. Tell them they can always ask for help and maybe keep the tasks they have to organise to a minimum, so they don't become overwhelmed. Remember, while it's good to encourage independence, there is no rush to for them to grow up or at least at the rate of NT children their age – it's not a competition.

- **Unable to sit still** – There are many sensory items available that can help with this such as weighted blankets, weighted vests, sensory toys, also proprioceptive exercises on the hands can help with sitting still for long. ND children (and adults) need movement breaks and downtime to regulate. If this does become a long-term issue affecting their health, OT support and medication can help.

- **Constantly fidgeting** – Advice same as above but if it isn't harmful to themselves or anyone else, is it really an issue? There may be times it's not appropriate, but if it helps the child concentrate (which it often will, like explained for stimming) in my opinion it's not a huge problem and something they may grow out of. ALL children naturally have more energy than adults anyway.

- **Excessive talking** – Something else that a lot of young children do, ND or NT, and something which most will grow out of as they mature. Of course, they need to learn when talking isn't appropriate so work on that first, which school should also help with.

- **Interrupts conversations** – Advice same as above and something that the child may have to work on for a very long time, but please teach them that it's how their brain works, they're not bad people so don't need to be embarrassed, and to just try their best and assure them that you will support them.

- **Unable to wait their turn** – Again, something ALL children need to learn and children with ADHD can learn this. You may need to repeat yourself many, many times, but practice makes perfect, and it is possible. Nobody really likes waiting but it can't be helped in some situations in life; try to reduce those situations where possible to prevent overwhelm or at least prepare them when you know it will be necessary.

- **Impulsive actions** – As the child matures, they will learn that there are consequences to their actions which will help if someone supportive can explain this to them. If it continues into adulthood and affects their health and/or daily life, therapy and medication can also help.

- **Little or no sense of danger** – Of course, this is worrying, but I think with any child, especially ND children, firstly, they should never be left alone in a situation where there are possible dangers. This is one of the hardest parts of having an ND child as they can mature slower than other children and seem younger for longer, and therefore you must continue to monitor them constantly which can be stressful, so this is why support and respite is vital for us parents. Always explain the reasons of why they must hold your hand in a car park, for example, or why they can't climb and jump from high spaces, and eventually they can and will learn with constant support.

- **Poor sleeping patterns** – This can be one of the hardest areas of parenting a child with ADHD and it's a vicious circle because children need sleep to develop and sustain attention, and the less sleep they get the harder it is. Sleep massively influences ADHD traits – the less sleep we get, the more tired we are and the more stressed we will get. We all NEED sleep, it's vital, so you really need to follow a strict bedtime routine such as lights down and low volume around two hours before, no TV or iPad etc two hours before, no drinks an hour or so before, or if necessary just sips, try not to send them to bed hungry but not too full either, no sugar several hours before, a comfortable bed with sensory-aware bedding and pyjamas, a warm bath, lavender oil – not too much – and deep pressure massage on their joints as they lie in bed. Keep things short and sweet when you leave the room. If a child is very upset or afraid, my advice would be to do what is best for your whole family to get sleep – it won't last forever. Also, you can speak to your child development centre who can give advice, support, and medication if necessary.

In older children/adults:

- **Carelessness** – It helps to write things down that you need to remember. Also, routine helps a lot. Try to keep your home environment/learning space as uncluttered as possible and be aware of dangers if you tend to trip or be clumsy often.

- **Lack of attention to detail** – this will often be the case in areas that the person is not interested in, so just remember to pay attention to detail in the areas that are vital such as driving and keeping safe.

- **Often starts new tasks before completing last one** – Making to-do lists really helps and organising jobs so you know what you have to do, now and next. Planning your time realistically is also very important so you don't get overwhelmed, and remember to take breaks.

- **Poor organisational skills** – Again, writing things down massively helps. Remember, you can always ask for help and maybe keep the things you have to organise to a minimum, so you don't become overwhelmed. Don't put too much pressure on yourself.

- **Inability to focus or prioritise** – Again, writing things down and organising tasks in order of priority helps a lot. As you age, if this is having a negative effect on your daily life, medication can really help with focus if necessary.

- **Often loses or misplaces things** – Try your best not to get frustrated and learn to write things down that you need to remember and have specific places for important items, so you don't lose them. Routine helps a lot.

- **Forgetfulness** – Truly, writing things down on a calendar or diary and keeping it somewhere you will see every day helps so much.

- **Restlessness** – This can be a hard one because it's a vicious circle of physically not being able to rest but lack of rest exacerbating ADHD symptoms. Medication can help but also daily guided meditation is very helpful. As is finding a TV show or film etc you are interested in that will physically make you sit and watch, which forces you to rest your mind and to focus on something other than your thoughts. Try to make sure you sleep well as this helps the brain rest, which is vital for those of us with ADHD. Exercise is good to burn energy; also limiting sugar and caffeine intake in your diet helps too.

- **Speaks out of turn or interrupts others** – This quite often cannot be helped at a younger age, and it is more of a case of the people around you are understanding; however, of course we all need to learn to try our best not to be rude, nasty, or inappropriate, and this comes with practice, support, and experience. Just try your best and don't worry too much.

- **Mood swings** – Remember, being ND is hard at times and we are only human, many of us struggle to control our emotions as explained previously. Therapy and medication can help if this doesn't improve with age and time. Also, guided meditation is beneficial, making sure you sleep well as people with ADHD particularly struggle with their mood and mental health if they have poor sleep. Exercise such as boxing is also good for releasing frustrations. I also recommend practising gratitude with a journal each day as a good way to stay positive.

- **Struggles with anxiety and/or depression** – This is highly likely at times for those with ADHD simply because it can be overwhelming and, without awareness and support, can feel unmanageable. Therapy is extremely helpful as can be medication, and general advice for mental health is applicable. Please see the Helpful Tips section.

- **Inability to deal with stress** – Managing stress for people with ADHD is especially hard because our body and mind feels stressed most of the time as it is, so extra stress often overwhelms us. Again, good sleep is important, guided meditation, planning time for rest, exercise, connecting with people socially, sharing problems helps, and sticking to a routine and writing things down.

- **Extreme impatience** – Nobody likes to wait or do things they don't want to do, but some manage better than others. Try not to put yourself in a position often where you will become impatient or frustrated. Therapy can help with this and medication too if it becomes a real problem in your daily life.

- **Takes risks such as driving dangerously** – This is a big reason many people with ADHD take medication because of course safety is number one. If your actions are dangerous, such as driving, I would advise against it until you find a way to manage this.

- **Displays OCD habits** – Being clean and liking things in their place can be a positive thing, also (as previously explained) following routines can be calming for ND people, and if it doesn't harm anyone, I don't think it's a problem; however, if it becomes too much and interferes with the way in which you live your life, therapy can help, as can medication.

- **Hyperactivity which can be physical, verbal, or emotional** – The hyperactive mind is, in my opinion, one of, if not the hardest, thing about having ADHD. Not being able to be physically calm and still and just altogether being on the go constantly is exhausting; however, using the calming tips previously explained above can help, as can medication.

- **Poor time management** – All that can be done is your best. If you know that this can be an issue for you and you continue to work on it, it is something some of us will have to live with and be aware of. Planning our time realistically and not taking too much on helps a lot.

- **Easily distracted** – Again, routine and writing things down helps with this so that the problem doesn't get worse when you are distracted and forget what you were originally doing, because that's another vicious circle. Sleeping well and exercise helps focus, as can medication if necessary.

- **Impulsivity** – Those with ADHD can find it hard to make well thought out decisions and act without thinking things through rationally. This is known to affect males with ADHD more detrimentally with actions such as excessive alcohol consumption, overspending and overeating. If you feel this is affecting your daily life, please speak to your GP or anyone else you feel you can confide in.

Trust me when I say our conditions frustrate us more than they could ever frustrate anyone else, but this is how our brain works, it is how we're made and we're doing our best with that. Many ND people feel guilt for who they are and what this means for their families, friends, partner etc. I have learned to believe in the importance of self-worth and being positive and thankful for who you are. Nobody's perfect and if you're truly doing all you can, to be kind, understanding and happy, then you should have peace of mind and be proud of who you are as an individual. Some people won't like or understand us, and some don't want to understand us, but don't let that affect you or who you are, it really is their problem not yours. Because of my heightened intuition (which many ND people have), I am overly aware of other people's opinions of me, which can be a blessing and a curse. I ALWAYS know what people's intentions are even if I don't show it and I'm a great judge of character.

The only reason ND people are seen as 'strange' is because they are **different** and there are more NT people on the planet than us, BUT that doesn't mean we're wrong. Different does not mean less, just because there are more of one group than another doesn't mean that the bigger group is superior, correct or should be held in a higher regard. ND people often think the way NT people behave can be pretty 'strange', but we have been made and expected, for generations, to try and fit in and act in ways that don't make sense to us. Surely, it's now time to just let us be ourselves? We may sometimes not see the world in the same way that NT people do, but what we do see and the ideas we have are things nobody else could, and that is a gift, and for that I'm glad to be **different.**

"I'm autistic, which means everyone around me has a disorder that makes them say things they don't mean, not care about structure, fail to hyperfocus on important topics, have unreliable memories, drop weird hints, and creepily stare into my eyeballs. So why do people say I'm the weird one? Because there's more of them than me."

Chris Bonello (details in Recommended Resources)

Why fit in when you were born to stand out?

Dr Seuss

Iconic Children's Author

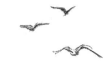

POSITIVE ASC AND ADHD TRAITS

Having a brain that works differently also GIVES us many skills and gifts that we can all learn to appreciate and be grateful for. Here are just some examples of the benefits we often have:

- Entrepreneurial abilities
- Intelligence
- Strong intuition
- Passionate
- Brave
- Persistence
- Resilience
- Thoughtful
- Happy in own company
- Good long-term memory
- Strong sense of injustice (for themselves and others)
- Self-awareness

- Independence
- Strength
- Honesty
- Loyalty
- Reliability
- High levels of empathy
- Deep thinkers
- The ability to hyper focus on special interests
- Tidiness
- Organisation
- Noticing and appreciating the small details in things
- Visual learners
- Unique thought processes/ideas
- Creativity
- Challenges opinions/social norms
- Strong willed
- Determination
- Accepting of other people's differences
- Not afraid to be themselves
- Confidence
- High energy
- Originality
- Great leadership skills
- Nonconformist
- Children/people on the spectrum are often super instinctive and great judges of character; I have always had this skill since I was very young. The fact

that we have to learn differently – and work hard to understand people and watch every detail – makes us experts on really seeing people and noticing non-verbal communication. There are many psychologists who are autistic as they can read people well due to the way in which they have studied them since childhood out of necessity. They can also better understand the way many of their clients who are ND think and behave.

There are many benefits
to adhd, too many
to list. It becomes a
disadvantage when you're
expected to conform to
a structure that doesn't
make sense to you.

Peter Carlisle

ADDitude Magazine

HOW TO BE HELPFUL TO NEURODIVERGENT PEOPLE

- Please don't use the word 'normal' when referring to NT people or mainstream schools etc.

- Do some research about what ASC/ADHD is, don't just expect us to have to educate you, and tell us you have done so; it feels good to know people have made the effort to understand us.

- Unless you're also ND you will never fully understand what it is like, but at least try and put yourselves in our shoes before you react or judge.

- Be patient when communicating with us, remember we sometimes need time to process what you've said and we don't always give good eye contact; this isn't us being rude.

- If we go off talking at length about something we're interested in this isn't us being selfish and we may just need some redirection back to the conversation. Be open with us, we appreciate that and understand that.

- Understand and appreciate that we like routine and schedules.

- Understand and appreciate that we're not usually fans of new places and if we are going to a new place, we may ask lots of questions first and want to do a lot of planning.

- Remember and appreciate that we can take things literally a lot of the time so may not understand certain jokes or slang.

- Some autistic people can overshare personal information; if you're not comfortable, try to change the subject to something more appropriate or kindly tell us you feel it's too personal to discuss. Again, we appreciate directness.

- Autistic people can struggle with boundaries; if you feel someone is too close, model how far away you feel is appropriate and if it doesn't stop just let them know. Remember what comes as natural to you often doesn't to us so help us learn.

- We may not wish (or be able) to communicate like you, for example I very rarely speak on the phone. I am much more comfortable to text or email and will often not answer a phone call. We all prefer to communicate in different ways; no way is right or wrong.

- Ask the person/parent if they are comfortable when you invite them somewhere or if you're out with them, to check if there's anything you could do to help such as dimming lights, reducing noise or turning your heating up. If we're not comfortable it can completely take our focus off enjoying our time with you.

- Don't assume a person's intellectual ability based on their diagnosis – being autistic or having ADHD does NOT mean unintelligent or less than; in fact, quite often the opposite!

- Simply ask the person how you can be a better friend, colleague, family member etc to them, we'll be happy to help you understand us.

- Try to help us socialise by including us in conversations with others.

- If you have NT children around a ND child, explain to them what their differences are, how we are all different, to be patient and kind and not to take it personally if they don't interact directly.

- Understand that plans need to be flexible – people with ASC may have a meltdown, shutdown or feel very anti-social for a number of reasons and should not be forced to do something we don't feel comfortable doing or be made to feel bad for cancelling. What may feel like a nice surprise to you could be the total opposite to someone who is autistic. If you must change plans, please give as much notice as possible, and if the person is upset or distressed give them time to calm down.

- Raising a ND child is a journey and things change, progress and evolve all the time, so check in to see how things are going like you would with anyone, but not in a 'are they talking yet?, are they eating sleeping alone yet?' way as this can be taken as condescending or negative if the child hasn't yet done these things; they may have had other positive progress and we as parents will be sure to tell you as we celebrate every little thing. We don't need extra pressure and don't always want to dwell on milestones etc.

- Remember it can be draining for us to socialise like NT people so we may need some quiet time or time alone away from others – don't think we're being rude.

- Remember and appreciate ND people really thrive with routine.

- Be specific with instructions to ND children, such as, "put your coat away" not "please can you go upstairs and hang your coat in the cupboard".

- Watch for warning signs, if you see a ND child becoming upset or overwhelmed take them away from the situation and let them have a break.

- Never take what you believe to be as rude/difficult behaviour personally, remember our brain works differently to those of most other people.

- Be open and honest, we love when people talk straight and we will do the same, so don't be offended, but let us know if this upsets you; don't just avoid us because we will have no clue what we did to offend you.

- Make the effort to check in/communicate with us – we often don't know what is appropriate.

- Don't think we don't want friendships or relationships, we do, we just find it more difficult than NT people and need people who make an effort and try to understand us.

- Don't just assume ASC/ADHD is something naughty kids have, or believe everything you've been told, and remember it's a hugely wide spectrum and what may affect one child/person may not affect the next. As the saying goes, **IF YOU'VE MET ONE PERSON WITH AUTISM THEN YOU'VE MET ONE PERSON WITH AUTISM.**

- If a child/person is non-verbal don't assume they can't hear you or understand you – they can, even if it doesn't look like it.

- Don't talk about them as if they're not there, they are.

- Don't talk about things in front of them that you wouldn't any other child.

- Don't assume they're of low intelligence, they're not.

- Include ND children in the conversation, it's good to follow their parent/carer's lead on this as they know them best.

- Pause after giving them directions/instructions etc to allow them to digest what has been said.

- Give them choices using pictures or visual aids such as 'pizza or spaghetti'. Don't make all their choices for them.

- Use visual schedules such as now and next.

- Ask the parent/carer how they like to communicate and if they use a device get to know how they use it.

- Always look at the person you're talking to, not their parent/carer.

- Use gestures when talking to them such as pointing to where they can hang their coat.

- Always communicate what you're doing even if they don't look interested.

- Talk to them like you do anyone else, maybe just slower and with more pauses; they don't want to be in silence.

- Always assume competence.

- Don't say "you don't look autistic", ASC has no influence on anyone's appearance, neither does ADHD.

- Don't say "you don't seem autistic" – prejudgement shows how little you know of our condition, and you need to learn more, this isn't a compliment to us!

- Don't say things like "my cousin is autistic so I know how it is", because just like NT people, all people on the spectrum are different; whilst there are some common traits we may share, we are not all the same, and living with ASC/ADHD or living with someone who has ASC/ADHD is very different to just knowing someone who has the condition.

- DO NOT say you're 'sorry' if we tell you our child is autistic or has ADHD or that you don't know how we "cope". Firstly, our child is nothing to be sorry for and secondly, we 'cope' just like every parent 'copes'.

- NOT EVERYONE IS ON THE SPECTRUM! DON'T SAY THEY ARE. It belittles the struggles those of us who actually are. YES, we ALL have our own ways and quirks, but that is completely different to having a neurological condition.

- Remember and appreciate, if we do something a different way to you or other NT people, it doesn't make it wrong, just different.

- Meltdowns or shutdowns occur in both autistic children and adults for a variety of reasons such as stress, being overwhelmed, being overstimulated, and whilst someone is in the middle of such a situation, please remember not to tell them off, not to be angry, not to criticise them, don't try to explain any consequences, don't demand something else from them and don't move them unless they are unsafe. Stay calm, don't panic, make sure they are safe, adjust the environment if needed such as reducing volume, lights, and other people. Wait for the episode to pass and be ready to support the recovery.

- Meltdowns or shutdowns are not a time to teach, not a time for conversation and they certainly aren't a choice from the sufferer. These times are not bad behaviour, they are a coping mechanism that our brain uses when we've had enough and should be understood and learned from to help reduce them.

- Really listen to what we're saying when we're communicating that we're struggling, we've often got to an overwhelmed stage if we're telling you.

- People with ADHD can sometimes take a long time to do a task – don't judge us for this or become angry. ADHD can be so debilitating at times that even simple tasks are too much. We procrastinate A LOT.

- Don't interrupt our line of conversation as we may forget what we were talking/thinking about which causes untold stress and repercussions.

- Focus on our strengths, don't point out our weaknesses as this can cause really low self-esteem; we already know what we find difficult and are doing our best.

- People with ADHD can be impulsive, they may not stop to consider the situation or consequences; you can provide guidance and show us what is sensible and safe.

- Give children with ADHD clear boundaries and praise positive behaviour so they know what is expected and what will not be tolerated. Discipline is very important.

Rarely, if ever, are any of us healed in isolation. Healing is an act of communion

Bell Hooks

Theorist, Professor and Author

TIPS ON HOW TO SUPPORT PARENTS OF CHILDREN WITH ASC/ADHD

- Include them and their children, we may have to say no a lot or cancel last minute, BUT we also need friends and a social life so be patient and don't take things personally. Also, our children may not interact with others the same as NT children do or be overwhelmed in certain situations, but at least ask so we the parent can decide, don't just assume. Autistic children often like being around other children (and it is good for them on both sides) even if it looks like they don't.

- Our families are not charity cases; connect with us genuinely and honestly like you do anyone else. Get to know us.

- Research when you have the time, about what ASC and/or ADHD is, don't just expect the parent to have to educate you, and tell them you have done so, it feels good to know people have made the effort to understand our family.

- Teaching your NT children about ND children will make them more understanding, kind adults in the future. Which makes the world a better place for EVERYONE.

- Do not judge, try to imagine what it would be like in their shoes. Being a parent is hard, being a parent to an autistic child and/or child with ADHD is harder a lot of the time, for many different reasons.

- If the parent chooses to discuss confidential matters about their child or parenting with you, please do keep it to yourself.

- Help parents by speaking up on their behalf, it's a gesture that won't be forgotten.

- Ask if there is anything you can do to help.

- Let them know you're there for them if they need to talk – you may not always know what they're going through, but you can always listen.

- Simply ask them how you can be a better friend, colleague, family member etc to them.

- Ask the child's parents what's the current thing you're working on? What can I talk to the child about? Get to know the child and understand them. Follow the parents' lead on routine, food, and behaviour.

- Offer to spend some time with the child to get to know them fully and when you do, maybe even ask if you could look after the child for a while so the parent can take a break and you can build a truly special relationship with a wonderful ND child.

- Tell the parents how much you admire the way they care for their child; positivity and praise are always a good thing and sometimes we need to hear it.

- If you are having a ND child in your home, ask the parent if there is anything specific they would like, and provide a quiet room in case the child needs to take a break.

- Don't assume their child is any less or question their intelligence – they're not.

- Treat us like you do everyone else, just understand our family may be a bit different to the 'norm'.

- Remember autistic children and children with ADHD, like all children, grow up, and what effort you put in now will be remembered by them when they're older and will likely shape their future.

- Know that our children can learn and do everything that EVERY child does, it just takes longer because of how their brain works and they may need to learn in a different way.

- Don't treat our children any differently to any other children, just understand their needs, they may have more/different ones than NT children – that's all.

We rise by lifting others

Robert G Ingersoll

Historical Campaigner, Lawyer, and Writer

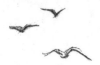

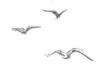

THE PROCESS
OF A CHILD
BEING DIAGNOSED

Please note this information is correct at the time of writing and may differ in your area. I write this with knowledge from the UK, practices differ greatly from country to country.

If, using any of the knowledge you have learned from this book, or any previous knowledge or thoughts you had, you believe your child could have ASC and/or ADHD, the following is the process for referral:

- If your child is below school age, you can advise your health visitor of your concerns and they will most likely visit your child and then start the referral process for assessment. You can also take your child to visit your GP and they will do the same.

- Health visitors really should pick up on any issues when they visit your child; however, due to staff shortages and high workloads this often isn't the case.

- If your child is of school age you can speak to their class teacher or ask to speak with the school SENCO (Special Education Needs Co-ordinator) who can make a referral for assessment. The teacher will usually have experience of these matters and will most likely have noticed signs within your child's behaviour as they spend a lot of time with them. You can also take your child to visit your GP and they will do the same.

- All schools and nurseries in the UK have their own assessment and referral process and they may pick up on any issues themselves which they will discuss with you; however, if not, you can start the process yourself.

- If you would prefer, and have the means, to go via the private route then please do your research and maybe even ask your GP if they can recommend a private clinic for assessments.

- REMEMBER unless you are lucky enough to be able to go via a private clinic there is a substantial wait for NHS assessments. It will be beneficial to your child's cause if you chase things up frequently and get personal contacts along the way who you can call or email directly. This will be a taste of the fight you will have if your child is diagnosed, unfortunately, but it is all of benefit to your child receiving the correct (and very much needed) help and support.

- Along the way expect to be asked to fill in many questionnaires about your child and to answer many repetitive questions – it's helpful to try and remember and give as much information as you can.

- Your child's teacher or health visitor will also be asked to give information.

- Your child will usually see a team of different specialists (either being observed in one day or separately) such as an OT, Educational Psychologist and Consultant Paediatrician, who will write reports.

- Any diagnosis due will be given, usually by a consultant paediatrician, using all these reports and information given as part of the process.

- REMEMBER if your child does receive a diagnosis you can apply for an EHCP which will help them get educational support. You can also apply for financial support to help with any special equipment or activities you need to support your child.

THE PROCESS
OF AN ADULT
BEING DIAGNOSED

Please note this information is correct at the time of writing and may differ in your area. I write this with knowledge from the UK, practices differ greatly from country to country.

If, using any of the knowledge you have learned from this book, or any previous knowledge or thoughts you had, you believe you could have ASC and/or ADHD the following is the process for referral:

- REMEMBER as an adult it is your responsibility to notice signs in your behaviour or functioning. You will need to be proactive in bringing this to the attention of your GP.

- If you have previously been diagnosed with a mental health condition and don't believe this is fitting, or at least that this isn't the root cause of your issues, visit your GP and make them aware. GPs often do not have the knowledge, or the time with patients, unfortunately, to proactively refer for assessments.

- If you would prefer, and have the means, to go via the private route then please do your research and maybe even ask your GP if they can recommend a private clinic for assessments.

- REMEMBER unless you are lucky enough to be able to go via a private clinic there is a substantial wait for NHS assessments. It will be beneficial to your cause if you chase things up frequently and get personal contacts along the way who you can call or email directly.

- As an adult you will be asked to fill in some questionnaires and some of your family who knew you when you were a child (if you have any) will also be asked to complete some; if not it is good if you can provide school reports but don't worry if not. Your partner/ spouse may also be asked for information about you.

- You will have quite an extensive 'interview' with an assessor – you will get breaks – where you will be asked lots of questions going right back to your childhood and back to the present day. Be prepared for this but not daunted. Remember this is a pathway to support.

- You may receive a diagnosis there and then or the assessor may need to get some specialist advice from their colleagues, or perhaps ask you to gather more information; if so a diagnosis or decision will be given in the not-too-distant future if needed.

Work harder on yourself than you do on your job

Jim Rohn

Motivational Speaker and Author

A FEW FACTS AND COMMON MYTHS REGARDING ASC AND ADHD

FACTS

- The earlier ASC/ADHD is diagnosed and treated, the better the outcome for children's lives being significantly improved.

- ASC/ADHD are not degenerative, meaning that ND individuals can continually progress with the right treatment and support.

- Being non-verbal as a child does not mean a person will never speak; research shows that many will learn to use words and nearly half will learn to speak fluently.

There are also many technologies that make it possible for non-verbal people to communicate. People can and do discover speech at any age.

- Approximately 70 million individuals have ASC worldwide – that we know of.

- A common coping strategy for people with ASC is repetitive behaviours often called 'stimming'. This can be repetitive body movements or a strong preference in sticking to routines.

- Food aversions are common in people with ASC mostly due to sensitivity to taste and texture.

- Meltdowns are a response to an overwhelmed brain, NOT a choice or bad behaviour.

- The average age of diagnosis in ADHD is currently seven years old.

- Having ASC/ADHD does not make a person less intelligent.

- ASC/ADHD symptoms can present differently at different times in people's lives.

- People with ADHD can often have hyperfocus which helps them to focus on a task or subject more intensely than NT people.

- ADHD can affect driving skills due to being less attentive and more impulsive.

- Untreated ADHD has more of a negative effect on a person's day-to-day life than those who are diagnosed and supported.

- In 1908, the word autism was first used by psychiatrist Dr Eugen Bleuler to describe a patient who had withdrawn into their own world. The Greek word autos means self.

- In 1943, Dr Leo Kanner diagnosed the first patient with ASC.

- IN 1902, Dr George Frederic Still described an abnormal deficit of control in children who could not control their behaviour.

- Originally ADHD was known as 'hyperkinetic reaction of childhood'.

- **Human progress depends on diversity of thought, we can't progress as a society with only one neurotype.**

MYTHS

- **ASC is caused by vaccines** – High quality research involving hundreds of thousands of people have consistently shown this not to be true. Also, there are many, many people with ASC that have never had a vaccine.

- **ASC/ADHD only affect children** – Both are lifelong conditions, and, in the UK, there are now actually more autistic adults than children.

- **All autistic people have a special talent** – All human beings have strengths and weaknesses, and autistic people are no different. However, due to the way our brain works, we often have intense interests and can focus on a subject more than those with a NT brain. Around 10% of autistic people show advanced levels of a particular skill.

- **Autistic people are anti-social** – Due to our condition, it can be difficult to build friendships and relationships as we communicate and think differently to NT people; however, that doesn't mean we don't want to have friends.

- **Autistic people are emotionless** – Differences in expression sometimes lead to this belief but, we have emotions even if you can't see them. In fact, recent research shows that we have an excess of empathy rather than a lack of it.

- **ASC/ADHD are learning disabilities** – These conditions are not learning disabilities but can affect the way in which we learn, and learning disabilities can coexist in people with ASC/ADHD.

- **Poor parenting causes ADHD** – A huge amount of research shows that social factors such as parenting do not contribute to the development of ADHD. It is a neurological condition; however, some parenting practices such as inconsistent discipline and low paternal involvement can worsen ADHD symptoms.

- **All people with ADHD are hyperactive** – This is a common stereotype, but ADHD mainly impacts attention, not hyperactivity at all. Many health professionals now use the term ADD instead of ADHD as there often is not hyperactivity.

Without deviation from the norm, progress is not possible.

Frank Zappa

Musician and Advocate

PEOPLE IN THE PUBLIC EYE WITH ASC OR ADHD

As you can see, these conditions do not have to hold you back in life or affect your success, in fact they can be a huge benefit!

ASC:

- Sir Anthony Hopkins – Actor
- Elon Musk – Entrepreneur (and richest man in the world)
- Daryl Hannah – Actress
- Dan Akroyd – Actor
- Wentworth Miller – Actor
- Sir Tim Burton – Film Director
- Satoshi Tajiri – Creator of Pokemon
- Woody Allen – Film Director

- Dr Temple Grandin – Animal Scientist, Author, and Autism Advocate
- Courtney Love – Actress

It is also widely believed that the following historical figures would now be diagnosed with ASC:

- Albert Einstein – Inventor
- Mozart – Music Composer
- Beethoven – Music Composer
- Leonardo da Vinci – Artist
- Henry Ford – Inventor
- Hans Christian Andersen – Author
- Lewis Carroll – Author
- Charles Darwin – Scientist
- Steve Jobs – Former CEO of Apple
- Andy Warhol – Artist

ADHD:

- Simone Biles – Olympic Gymnast
- Emma Watson – Actress
- Johnny Depp – Actor
- Channing Tatum – Actor
- Justin Timberlake – Musician
- Dave Grohl – Musician

- Michael Phelps – Olympic Swimmer
- Solange Knowles – Musician (and sister of Beyonce)
- Tim Howard – Footballer
- Will.I.Am – Musician
- Adam Levine – Musician
- Zooey Deschanel – Actress
- Michelle Rodriguez – Actress
- Woody Harrelson – Actor
- Ryan Gosling – Actor
- Will Smith – Actor
- Jim Carrey – Actor
- Cameron Diaz – Actress
- Megan Fox – Actress
- Justin Bieber – Singer
- Paris Hilton – DJ/Reality Star/Entrepreneur

It is also widely believed that the following historical figures would now be diagnosed with ADHD:

- Vincent Van Gogh – Artist
- Pablo Picasso – Artist
- Benjamin Franklin – Inventor
- John Lennon – Musician
- Elvis Presley – Musician
- Steven Hawking – Scientist
- Muhammad Ali – Boxing Legend

What would happen if the autism gene was eliminated from the gene pool?
You would have a bunch of people standing around in a cave, chatting and socialsing and not getting anything done.

Dr. Temple Grandin

Inspirational Author and Autism Advocate

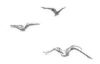

EPILOGUE

I f I can leave one message to my ND peers, it is this – ALWAYS BE YOURSELF.

Be proud of who you are and don't apologise for it. Comparison is the root of unhappiness for ANYONE and EVERYONE. Don't worry about what anyone else's life looks like or what anyone else's idea of happiness is. Find your own happiness, find the life that YOU want, and make it happen.

My biggest hope (and I truly believe it will happen) is that ND people around the world are accepted for who they are, and that any stigma or negativity surrounding ASC and ADHD disappears. That is how it can be, that is how it should be, and it will create a better world for us ALL.

It isn't just people who are inexperienced that hold the beliefs that limit ND children and adults, you would be surprised at the amount of 'professionals', whose job it is to work with us, who have no idea of our potential or what is best for us. For example, a fellow parent of mine, who has a young autistic son who is non-verbal, was recently told by a support worker (who has for many years, and still does, work with autistic children for a living) that their family should accept that they simply can't take him on family days out. This is nonsense. The child is five years old and is still learning, as are his family, and he has been involved in many trips, days out and holidays, that, although can look 'different' to some others, have been enjoyable for all involved. With experience, maturity, confidence, and continued support, this will only continue and enhance his life and that of his family. We may need to plan things out in more detail, be less spontaneous and make some allowances, but autistic children and/or children with ADHD can absolutely enjoy the same things that others do, if they so wish.

The bigger picture is that EVERY person who works with children should be trained in all aspects of ASC and ADHD and trained by people who understand the conditions properly. Also, anyone who works with or cares for adults with ASC and/or ADHD should be adequately trained to understand their needs. This training will need to be ongoing and updated accordingly as we learn more as the years go by. It is a huge issue for families of ND children that the provision and support often abruptly end when someone turns 18. As I have mentioned, our conditions are lifelong so don't just go away once we reach adulthood, and those who struggle more than others will still need education and support. The current provision for this is not good enough and is something that many parents continue to campaign for.

Breaking the outdated stigma and stereotypes that many people have, and supporting the ND community, will only help our society in the long run – it's quite simple.

This topic is a huge part of my life and something I am passionate about and love to keep learning about. You will see on the final page the address for my new Instagram page in which I am hoping to build a community in which myself and others can share experiences, advice, support, and inspiration.

The start to a better world is a belief that it's possible.

Norman Cousins

Author, Professor and World Peace Advocate

RECOMMENDED RESOURCES

All the below I have read, followed, and watched over the several years since my son was diagnosed, and during my own journey, which have all helped me immensely.

WEBSITES

WWW.AUTISM.ORG.UK

This is the website for the National Autistic Society which is arguably the largest ASC charity in the UK. There is a huge amount of information for EVERYONE here. This is also home to a popular online forum for ND people.

WWW.AMBITIOUSABOUTAUTISM.ORG.UK

Another great ASC charity which you may find helpful.

WWW.NHS.UK/AUTISM AND WWW.NHS.UK/CONDITIONS/ATTENTION-DEFICIT-HYPERACTIVITY-DISORDER-ADHD/DIAGNOSIS/

This will take you directly to all the current information the NHS provide on ASC and ADHD.

WWW.ADHDUK.CO.UK

This charity was set up by people with ADHD, for people with ADHD, and their families, and is the most well known in the UK.

WWW.MIND.ORG.UK/ADHD

Mind is a large mental health charity, and this is the web address for their information on ADHD. They also hold some useful information on ASC as well as support forums.

WWW.SCOPE.ORG.UK

Scope is a charity for ALL disabilities, and their website holds a lot of information covering a huge range of topics. They also have a popular online forum for ND people to communicate.

INSTAGRAM PAGES

@NATIONALAUTISTICSOCIETY

This is the Instagram page for the charity above which highlights personal stories and important events.

@AUTISMPARENTINGMAGAZINE
This Instagram page from the Autism Parenting Magazine shares some popular memes for parents of children with ASC and you can also access their magazine.

@ADHDUK.CO.UK
This is the Instagram page for the charity above and shares some very useful information with regards to their online support groups and in-person advice clinics.

@AUTISTICNOTWEIRD
This is a personal favourite of mine and is owned by Chris Bonnello, who is an adult with ASC who shares his views, experiences, and a lot of information that he has learned – often in a very humorous way.

@DOC_AMEN
The page for Dr Amen whose books I recommend – he provides lots of good advice here.

@STORIESABOUTAUTISM
This is a popular account run by James who is a single co-parenting dad to two non-verbal boys with ASC. The page is very real and relatable to a lot of parents with children on the spectrum.

@AUTISTICPROFESSIONALSPEAKER

This account is run by Kerry Magro, who is an adult on the spectrum who now advocates for ASC via professional speaking. He has also written a few books, one of which is listed further below. Kerry has also consulted for autistic characters on several TV shows and films. He certainly proves that ASC doesn't need to hold you back!

@NEURODIVERGENT_LOU

I love this page as it shares A LOT of practical information and relatable opinions from a young adult with ASC.

@MYLADYADHD

This account is run by ADHD advocate Trina Hayes and shares a lot of useful and practical tips/advice for people with ADHD.

@STEVEN

This account is owned by Steven Bartlett who is the successful young entrepreneur who now appears on the TV show Dragon's Den. Steven shares many inspiring stories with his podcast 'The Diary Of A CEO'. This page is not directly related to ASC or ADHD, but I find that it highlights the importance of personal wellbeing, positivity and it does frequently discuss mental health issues which many of us with these conditions can struggle with.

@THEFUNNYMOMMA

Katryce who is a 'proud mom to a little on the spectrum' shares stories, videos, and inspiration that other ND parents may find positive and relatable for their own journey.

BOOKS

TEN THINGS EVERY CHILD WITH AUTISM WISHES YOU KNEW – ELLEN NOTBOHM

I found this book when I was at the beginning of our ASC journey with Jude, and it was so helpful that I ordered it for all our family to read to get an insight into the condition without being too complicated. My number one recommendation for anyone with an autistic child and their families/friends.

MORE THAN WORDS – FERN SUSSMAN (HANEN COMMUNICATION TECHNIQUES)

Invaluable advice for parents with children who are non-verbal or have limited speech. This would be my first port of call for you and my number one recommendation for those parents of children with communication issues.

HEALING ADD – DR DANIEL G AMEN

As I've mentioned, Dr Amen's knowledge has been hugely educational and inspiring for me personally and

I would recommend everyone who is interested in this area to read his books. They are full of knowledge and advice that can genuinely improve the life of those with ADHD alongside general brain health tips that are great for everyone.

DEFINING AUTISM FROM THE HEART – BY KERRY MAGRO

An inspiring true story by Kerry from the US who is now an adult with ASC detailing his childhood and growing up on the spectrum and how loving, supportive parents can help their children achieve anything.

THE AUTISTIC BRAIN – BY DR TEMPLE GRANDIN

Temple is a truly inspirational lady with ASC who has lived an extraordinary life and now advocates for those on the spectrum. As one of the first people to discuss ASC openly, she has changed the autistic world for the better for many. She has written several books (another one is listed below, and I have also recommended the film about her life further below).

THE WAY I SEE IT – BY TEMPLE GRANDIN

Temple writes about the real issues that people on the spectrum face as well as their parents. She offers a lot of helpful advice and information which has been updated over the years.

SINCERELY YOUR AUTISTIC CHILD – EDITED BY MORENIKE GIWA ONAIWU, EMILY PAIGE BALLOU AND SHARON DAVANPORT

This is a series of quotes and short stories written by young people with ASC detailing what they wish their parents had known when they were growing up. Well worth a read for parents of autistic children.

THE REASON I JUMP – BY NAOKI HIGASHIDA

This is a beautiful story written by Naoki when he was just 13 years old. Naoki describes what life is like for a non-verbal child/person **in his experience** and it is a wonderful insight into his world. This story has also been made into an award-winning film which some may find uncomfortable, or totally unrelatable to their child or their own journey, but if you would like to widen your learning it's worth a watch.

TENDER: THE IMPERFECT ART OF CARING – BY PENNY WINCER

This is an honest book which teaches us the important lesson of caring for ourselves when we care for others, a good read for parents/carers of people with ASC/ADHD.

A BEGINNER'S GUIDE ON PARENTING CHILDREN WITH ADHD – BY VIVIAN FOSTER

This book offers a wide range of helpful advice and information for parents of children, now and as they grow, with ADHD, and is definitely worth a read.

TAKING CHARGE OF ADHD IN ADULTS THE SILENT STRUGGLE – BY L.WILLIAM ROSS

This is a great book for adults with ADHD who want to learn more about their condition, how to accept ADHD and how to live your life to the fullest.

MANIFEST – BY ROXIE NAFOUSI

This book is not related directly to either condition; however, I found that its words and moral were very inspiring for those who are looking for a guide in positivity and self-awareness, which many ND people do.

TV PROGRAMMES/FILMS

INSIDE OUR AUTISTIC MINDS – AVAILABLE ON BBC IPLAYER

This documentary created by long standing TV presenter Chris Packham (Chris himself has ASC and shared this publicly a few years ago) is quite frankly the best I have seen regarding the condition so far with regards to autistic adults. In the two-part programme Chris meets several people who are on the spectrum and delves into their lives in a very realistic and informative way. The subjects explain and show how it feels to be autistic and it is particularly poignant when a non-verbal young man communicates his intelligence and the frustration he feels at not being able to speak. I am super thankful to Chris for using his platform and resources to make this programme and his continued advocacy. I would recommend EVERYONE to watch.

TANYA BARDSLEY (ME AND ADHD) – AVAILABLE ON ITV
This is a one-off programme in which reality star and TV personality Tanya openly discusses her ADHD diagnosis (which she received just before turning 40) and how the condition has and does affect her life. Tanya speaks to several others in the show such as the charity ADHDUK and parents of children with ADHD.

EVERYTHING'S GONNA BE OKAY – AVAILABLE ON DISNEY PLUS
This is a TV series which explores the family dynamics of someone with ASC during the ups and downs of life. I think representation of ND is always worth a watch.

LOOP – AVAILABLE ON DISNEY PLUS

By Disney, this is a beautiful animated short film with a non-verbal lead character which has a positive message.

HEARTBREAK HIGH – AVAILABLE ON NETFLIX

A Netflix remake of an Australian TV series featuring a young autistic character (in real life and on screen) unlike anything else currently shown. It is a relatable representation for young adults in the modern world. Award winning Chloe Hayden plays Quinni and is a huge advocate for ND with her writing and social media.

AS WE SEE IT – AVAILABLE ON AMAZON PRIME

I really enjoyed this series which features three unfiltered main autistic characters (played by people with ASC which is a joy in itself!). With the help of an assistant, they move in together as their parents are keen for them to become more independent. It is emotional at times but inspiring for many different reasons.

ATYPICAL – NETFLIX

This show is a comedy revolving around the autistic character Sam, who as a young adult has decided he is ready for a romantic relationship.

THE GOOD DOCTOR – NETFLIX

This is a popular series featuring well known actor Freddie Highmore as Shaun, who is a young adult with ASC. Shaun is a newly qualified doctor whose condition allows him to excel in his chosen career.

TEMPLE GRANDIN – AVAILABLE ON AMAZON PRIME

This film details the life story of Dr Temple Grandin. Temple is played by hugely popular actress Claire Danes and is definitely worth a watch.

THE A WORD – AVAILABLE ON BBC

This was the first show I watched that featured an autistic character and I think it does a good job of portraying how having a child with ASC affects the whole family, and in particular the relationship of the parents. The young actor, Max Vento, who plays the lead character Joe is not autistic in real life, but he does a great job in my opinion. The series features many successful British actors such as Christopher Ecclestone.

LIFE, ANIMATED – AVAIALBLE ON AMAZON PRIME

This heart-warming film is a real-life documentary which follows Owen Suskind, who has ASC, and his family. Owen suddenly stopped speaking as a toddler and didn't regain speech for several years, and in this film, he shows how his interest in certain TV characters helped him verbalise and communicate with his family.

EUPHORIA – AVAILABLE ON AMAZON PRIME

This series is not directly related to ASC or ADHD, and I must point out that it is NOT for children's viewing – parts of the show are graphic and quite sexual (the plot revolves around a group of young adults/teenagers and their relationships). However, the main character Rue, breathtakingly played by young award-winning actress Zendaya, has mental health problems (ADHD is mentioned when she is assessed as a young child) and a drug addiction. A lot of Rue's dialogue, particularly in conversation with her NA sponsor, relates to living with ADHD and how/why many people with the condition use alcohol and/or drugs to self-medicate.

Rue is 17 years old and has known she is 'different' her entire life which is difficult, and the show explores her learning how to live with such issues and how it also affects her family and friends.

Euphoria was created by Sam Levinson who uses his own experiences with drug addiction as a teenager and young adult to tell Rue's story.

BOOKS TO READ TO/ WITH YOUR CHIDREN

- I AM ENOUGH – GRACE BYERS
- THE BOY, THE MOLE, THE FOX AND THE HORSE – CHARLIE MACKESY
- INCREDIBLE YOU – RHYS BRISENDEN AND NATHAN REED
- HOW TO CATCH A STAR – OLIVER JEFFERS
- OH, THE PLACES YOU'LL GO! – DR SEUSS
- DIFFERENT A GREAT THING TO BE! – HEATHER AVIS AND SARAH MENSINGA
- MY MONSTER AND ME – NADIYA HUSSAIN AND ELLA BAILEY
- ONLY ONE YOU – LINDA KRANZ
- THE LION INSIDE – RACHEL BRIGHT AND JIM FIELD
- THE LAST BEDTIME STORY THAT WE READ EACH NIGHT – CAROL GRAY
- HOW ARE YOU FEELING TODAY – MOLLY POTTER
- STARTING SCHOOL – JANET AND ALLAN AHLBERG

REFERENCES/
BIBLIOGRAPHY

In addition to the knowledge I have gained from my personal experiences over the years, the below websites have also been used for research purposes in writing this book.

WWW.AUTISM.ORG.UK – September 2022

WWW.ADHDUK.CO.UK – October 2022

WWW.AMAZON.CO.UK – November 2022

WWW.WIKIPEDIA.COM – November 2022

WWW.NHS.UK – November 2022

WWW.NEWS-MEDICAL.NET – October 2022

WWW.NCBI.NLM.NIH.GOV – October 2022

WWW.SPECTRUMNEWS.ORG – November 2022

WWW.HEALTHLINE.COM – October 2022

WWW.RANKER.COM – November 2022

WWW.ADDITUDEMAG.COM – October 2022

WWW.LIFESPAN.ORG – November 2022

WWW.ADD.ORG – November 2022

WWW.CDC.ORG – November 2022

WWW.MASSGENERAL.ORG – November 2022

WWW.NATIONALAUTISMASSOCIATION – November 2022

WWW.SOMEONESMUM.CO.UK – November 2022

WWW.THESPECTRUM.ORG.AU – November 2022

WWW.MIND.ORG.UK – March 2023

WWW.GOV.UK – March 2023

WWW.AMENCLINICS.COM – November 2023

ABOUT THE AUTHOR

Jessica lives in the Northwest of England, with her husband Shaun and son Jude.

Jessica was diagnosed with ASC and ADHD, separately, in 2022 at the age of 38.

Jude is currently non-verbal and was diagnosed with ASC in 2018 and ADHD in 2023.

The three of them enjoy a quiet life together.

Jessica has always had a talent for writing from a young age and has a huge passion for reading, particularly non-fiction and criminal psychology.

She also loves to travel, enjoys fashion and food!

With some of her spare time, Jessica enjoys collecting and organising for local charities, particularly those that help the homeless and disadvantaged children, alongside continuously learning and advocating for those with ASC and ADHD.

Instagram: *@_theaalife_*
Website: *www.theautisticmom.net*
Email: *info@theautisticmom.net*

If you don't
like the road
you're walking,
start paving
another one

Dolly Parton